THE DEVIL AND DR. FAUCI:

The Many Faces of Bureaucratic Evil

James P. Driscoll, Ph.D.,

THE DEVIL AND DR. FAUCI:

The Many Faces of Bureaucratic Evil

James P. Driscoll, Ph.D.,

Academica Press
Washington~London

Library of Congress Cataloging-in-Publication Data

Names: Driscoll, James P. (author)
Title: The devil and dr. fauci : the many faces of bureaucratic evil | Driscoll, James P.
Description: Washington : Academica Press, 2021. | Includes references.
Identifiers: LCCN 2021947822 | ISBN 978-1680537475 (hardcover) | 978-1680537482 (paperback) | 9781680537499 (e-book)

Contents

BOOKS BY JAMES P. DRISCOLL

IDENTITY IN SHAKESPEAREAN DRAMA

THE UNFOLDING GOD OF JUNG AND MILTON

SHAKESPEARE & JUNG: THE GOD IN TIME

SHAKESPEARE'S IDENTITIES

JUNG'S CARTOGRAPHY OF THE PSYCHE

HOW AIDS ACTIVISTS CHALLENGED AMERICA,
And Saved FDA from Itself.

THE DEVIL AND DR. FAUCI:
The Many Faces of Bureaucratic Evil

Forthcoming.
CARL VERSUS KARL: Jung and Marx, Two Icons for our Age

Acknowledgements

First, I want to thank Paul du Quenoy, publisher of Academica Press, for offering to bring out an unusual and what may well prove to be a controversial work. Let me thank some of the people who gave me readers' feedback including Bill Arnold, Victoria Alexander, Karen Bak, Glinda Dignam, Edson Donovan, Paul Kainen, Felix Martel, and Ed Williams. Special thanks to Ed Williams for his "updating" the cover image, which he open sourced from its owner, the Wellcome Foundation, whom I thank for making their marvelous image freely available to all. As an American citizen, I want to salute former President Donald Trump for his heroic leadership in pushing the Covid 19 vaccines in record time through our too often dilatory FDA. Against great obstacles and much unfair criticism, he acted wisely and forcefully to save countless lives and restore our economy. I'd also like to commend Senators Rand Paul and Ron Johnson, two lonely voices of integrity crying out in the wilderness of the Washington Swamp. Lastly, I want to acknowledge my Bengal cat, Ariel, who gave me his devoted company sitting patiently on my desk while I labored on this work amidst the enforced isolation of the Covid pandemic.

The reader will encounter herein scientific and medical information about Covid 19, an extremely current, vital, and controversial subject. Although I have made every effort to be accurate, no one should make medical decisions based on this work without first consulting with their physicians. My opinions, political, philosophical, medical, and otherwise, are my own, not those of Academica Press.

Introduction

Onkel (Jung) said that the Germans were in league with the devil and had a lust for power which is Satanic. Onkel then went on to say that the Germans were Faust in his pact with the Devil.[1]

To compare Dr. Anthony Fauci with the Dr. Faustus of medieval lore, or with the hero of Christopher Marlowe's play, or the protagonist of Goethe's epic poem, may at first seem odd. The Faustus of lore and literature seems more richly complex and intriguing, and more likable than the egocentric contemporary American uber-bureaucrat with a similar name. Yet there are parallels for which Jung's remark offers illumination. Among them is the shared lust to possess the black magic of power, fame, and forbidden knowledge which draws the over-reaching Dr. Johann Faust to Mephistopheles and characterizes Dr. Anthony Fauci's attraction to dangerous Chinese gain of function virus research. Like the medieval Faustus, Fauci manifests the over-reacher archetype with its deep roots in myth and legend going back to trickster figures, shape shifters, and ultimately the Biblical Nimrod, the first great bureaucratic empire builder who started the Tower of Babel.

Being Swiss German himself, Jung located the Satanic power drive too exclusively in the Germans who carried part of the shadow of the Swiss. Jung identified a symptom of the German problem but overlooked its enabling cause, arrogant, unaccountable bureaucracies. The Germans decisive flaw was not so much love of power as an obsession with order that led them to rely on and implicitly trust Prussian style bureaucracy thereby blinding them to its great potential for facilitating amorality and outright evil. Without the German's trust of bureaucratic order embodied in Adolf Eichmann's "we were just following orders" ethic, the evils of Auschwitz would never have been possible, nor Himmler's SS, nor even Hitler's war machine. And that takes us to Dr. Anthony S. Fauci, kingpin of the ***Drug Licensing, Testing and Marketing Complex*** that runs America's war against the Covid 19 pandemic, and, as of this writing, still enjoys the blind, unmerited trust of the naïve majority of the American people.

We can thank the Covid 19 virus for giving the entire world a powerful, if implicit, warning on the pressing dangers and endemic evils of modern bureaucracy. Evidently bred of carelessness or possibly malign intent during gain of function research at the Wuhan Institute of Virology, the Covid virus has demonstrated to the world the needs for more vigilant oversight and stricter accountability on our increasingly powerful and too often rogue bureaucracies. Though the early lessons from the Nazis and Soviets were incisively drawn by George Orwell, Hannah Arendt, Alexander Solzhenitsyn and others, they have been largely forgotten by an indolent Western populace that knows almost nothing of its own recent history and has become accustomed to getting information in sound bites. Moreover, they are ignored by our neo-Marxist academia and media that mistakes parroting talking points for thinking. While the pandemic constantly reminds us of the hazards of trusting modern bureaucracies, the task of learning and applying its lessons has scarcely begun.

To understand the multifarious havoc Covid 19 has wrought in the US, in other Western democracies, and across the globe, we must first recognize what, I suspect, may currently be the most serious single internal threat to the survival of our democracy, our freedoms, and possibly of ourselves: the ***DTLM or the Drug Testing, Licensing, and Marketing Complex*** that controls, with close to zero effective outside oversight, the drug, biotech, vaccine, and medical devices research, development, licensing and marketing in the US and much of the world.

President Eisenhower, in his January 17, 1961 Farewell Address famously warned against the power of the ***Military Industrial Complex***. Ike is credited with alerting the nation to a danger that otherwise might have been dismissed as another crank conspiracy theory had the warning come from a less knowledgeable voice. No Eisenhower has stepped forward to warn us against the self-serving excesses and our dangerously deficient oversight on the Drug Testing, Licensing, and Marketing Complex. President Trump might have challenged this lurking devil and perhaps he still could, but, in respect to general credibility and public trust, Trump is not Eisenhower.

During the Covid 19 pandemic the DTLM Complex has proven to be every bit as powerful, refractory, and deviously self-serving as the Military Industrial Complex in its heyday of the Cold War. Both complexes stealthily maneuver to manipulate situations and facts, thereby relegating elected officials to dumbly accepting their decisions as *fait accompli*. The general public, popular culture, media, and the political sphere, however, have yet to recognize the cunning powers of the DTLM devil or our deficient oversight on it and the dangers inherent in its lack of accountability. In fact, the healthcare industry, which the DTLM Complex largely controls, is, at 18% of GDP, 5 times larger than our national defense budget at 3.4% of GDP. In 1961, when Eisenhower left office, healthcare was a mere 5% of GDP; defense stood at 6% of GDP. Spurring this trend, increasing percentages of our aging population have become ever more dependent on the products and services of the DTLM just to stay alive, your author is among these vulnerable dependents.

The Military-Industrial Complex led us into destructive, and what many believe were largely unnecessary wars in Vietnam, Iraq, and Afghanistan, and it encouraged us to focus on the mono-menace of Russia at the expense of ignoring other serious perils such as the ascension of China and Jihadist Islam. In this effort, they have been joined by their quietly rising replacement, the DTLM Complex whose corporations profit lavishly from trade with China. Indeed, the threats from the Military-Industrial Complex and the DTLM Complex are domestic parallels to the threats from the old Soviet Union and the new CCP China.

A major difference between the Military-Industrial Complex and the DTLM is that the former had no long term leader to symbolize its power and inflated attitudes, except cinema villains like General Jack Ripper from Stanley Kubrick's 1964 black comedy *Dr. Strangelove*. The DTLM has the real life Dr. Anthony S. Fauci, who is the iconic manifestation of the Dr. Johann Faustus archetype for our frenzied, chaotic, science worshipping era. Dr. Fauci gained world fame by becoming the spokesman and symbol of misguided, erratic US Covid policies which most Western oriented countries pursued like rats following Fauci playing Pied Piper. The hastily launched, destructive lockdowns without regard to collateral damage, the carnival posturing with problematic masks, the sole reliance on the black magic of hi-tech solutions, especially vaccines, while rejecting existing low-tech, low cost remedies to prevent or treat Covid, these were all championed by Dr. Fauci and his DTLM Complex cronies at the FDA, NIH, and CDC. As the most prominent architect and advocate of these crippling policies, Anthony S. Fauci is also a key author of the national and worldwide socio-economic devastation in the wake of their limitations and failures.

Extremely high risk gain of function research and vaccine technology represent for Dr. Anthony Fauci the black magic for which the medieval and literary Dr. Johann Faust sold his soul to the demon Mephistopheles. Finding viable vaccines for Covid was and remains a good and necessary objective which I support fully. But sole reliance on a vaccine solution is a dangerously restrictive strategy, particularly when numerous reputable clinicians in the field believe they have found prophylaxis and treatment options that, if used systematically, could bring major reductions in the toll from Covid. But we do not use them widely because Dr. Fauci, the FDA, and the DTLM Complex decided they might interfere with their own prioritization of and profits from Covid vaccines. It was as if Franklin D. Roosevelt had decided not to invade Normandy or defend Australia and Hawaii from the Japanese, he would just wait for Robert Oppenheimer to hand him atomic bombs to nuke Hiroshima and Berlin. Maybe that would have saved the trouble and expense of our war build up, but think of the cost in human suffering of letting the armies of Hitler and Hirohito ravage Europe and Asia for several more death filled years.

Some will object that I have written a book that is highly critical of scientists, especially Dr. Fauci, but am not a scientist myself. Why, they may ask, is a literary critic and a scholar who has written books on Shakespeare, Milton, and Carl Jung venturing into this area so removed from his expertise? First, let me note that understanding Shakespeare, Milton, and Jung is excellent preparation for fathoming anything that humans do. But also, the science on Covid and corona viruses is far from being settled: criticizing Fauci's off the cuff opinions is not comparable to criticizing Newton's laws of motion. Moreover, I've taken care to insure that my specific criticisms of Dr. Fauci have first been made by distinguished scientists in their fields. I do not rely exclusively on my own judgments. Third, where science has huge medical, economic, political and social implications the views of scientists need oversight from educated perspectives outside of science, including from religion, philosophy, history, psychology, and literature. Finally, I have a unique perspective which joins my broad understanding of these humanistic subjects with three decades of experience as a prominent FDA reform, AIDS, and LGBT rights activist. It is my hope that my multi-perspective critique of Fauci, the DTLM Complex, and the FDA may spark other non-scientists to apply their unique backgrounds and experiences to understanding the entire Covid pandemic.

Fauci, the FDA, and the DTLM Complex often appear to suffer from what Carl Jung might have seen as a peculiarly modern inflation: the imbalanced obsession with high tech final solutions at the expense of low tech limited or partial solutions. In such, they are driven by attitudes, typical of the Faustian archetype, that in our time moves us to blindly worship science and technology and seek in them a panacea for all problems. Thus, it is not black magic but the inflated promises of high tech that the contemporary devil uses to tempt over-reachers, of which Dr. Anthony Fauci is currently our most salient example. Yet Fauci and his DTLM cronies would get nowhere were they not enabled by the devil's most insidious modern heresy, the totalitarian bureaucrats' Adolf Eichmann credo-excuse of "only following orders."

Some of what ensues, especially the treatment of Tony Fauci himself, may seem satiric: that's because it deliberately is. Often the best way to get people to seriously examine intimidating public figures and scrutinize troubling social and political movements is to highlight their absurd aspects by making them laughable. Charlie Chaplin may have done a better job educating the public about Hitler than did any of our political leaders. Showing folly and evil as laughable disarms them, thereby empowering people to recognize what's bad and then moving them to reject and replace it. So far the public has not done that with Dr. Fauci and his familiar devils, the FDA and the DTLM Complex, or the myths and illusions they have concocted to empower and sustain them.

Thus, we have with Dr. Fauci, the FDA, and the DTLM Complex an "emperor's new clothes" situation. My objective in writing this short book is to open the eyes of its readers to these three "emperor's" nakedly self-serving deeds, motives, and modus operandi. Only by dispelling the illusions that blind us can we find our way to make life and soul saving reforms.

Chapter 1

The DTLM Devil and Dr. Fauci

Attacks on me are, quite frankly, attacks on science
—Dr. Anthony S. Fauci

America and the world have yet to fully experience, let alone grasp, the magnitude of the overall damage to our economy, society, and possibly our democratic freedoms, inflicted by the Covid 19 crisis. That damage continues to be aggravated by incompetent, irresponsible, self-serving DTLM Complex bureaucrats. Collateral damage to the US and the world from draconic lockdowns to combat Covid will exceed the human and financial costs of the Vietnam and the Iraq wars combined. For example, the CDC has reported an unprecedented drop in US life expectancy:

> *As the Covid-19 pandemic took hold, life expectancy in the U.S. dropped one full year during the first half of 2020 . . . Life expectancy at birth for the total U.S. population declined from 78.8 years in 2019 to 77.8 years for January through June 2020. During that same time period, life expectancy for non-Hispanic Black people decreased by 2.7 years (74.7 to 72); for Hispanics, 1.9 years (81,8 to 79,9) and for non-Hispanic white people, 0.8 years (78.8 to 78).*[2]

A one-year decline in US life expectancy, were it permanent, approximates the loss of 4 million lives, with African-Americans and other minorities suffering disproportionately. Yet so far 740,000 Americans have died with Covid, the additional deaths were collateral damage from Covid through suicide, drug and alcohol abuse, despair at financial set-backs and social isolation, and from failure to get medical care for other urgent ailments like cancer. During the lockdowns:

> *46% of the most common cancers were not diagnosed. 85% of living organ donor transplants were not done. Two thirds of cancer screenings were not done. Half of the 650,000 people on chemotherapy did not come in for their chemo. Half of our immunizations did not get done.*[3]

Besides all the added deaths, the US birthrate collapsed, reflecting the epidemic of frustration, isolation, doubt, and despair that has gripped our nation.

Many of the deaths were the largely avoidable results of lockdown overkill sanctioned and promoted by the DTLM Complex and its political allies. The chief DTLM spokesman and its leader has long been the recently ubiquitous Dr. Anthony Fauci. Fauci, whom Covid has elevated to become our society's iconic Big Brother figure, has headed the National Institute of Allergies and Infectious Diseases (NIAID) almost as long as J. Edgar Hoover, the first American icon of Big Brother, headed the FBI.

Although Dr. Fauci is a household name, before Covid he was little known beyond the beltway, except in the HIV-AIDS community. As strategist and spokesman for the US Covid response and *de facto* leader of the DTLM, Fauci's power for the long months of the lockdowns at times seemed to rival our nation's supreme military commanders during wartime. To the uncritical he appeared to be our U.S Grant or George Marshall. But actually he more resembles General William Tecumseh Sherman, in that, like Sherman, Fauci never allows himself to falter over the collateral damage from his unswerving martial campaigns. In Fauci's case, these campaigns involve mandatory masking, compulsory lockdowns, universal vaccination, and Orwellian suppression by cover up or censorship of opposing or alternative medical options and strategies. Beyond these, Fauci has attempted to suppress information about the origins of the Covid virus and about his own role in research that may have created it.

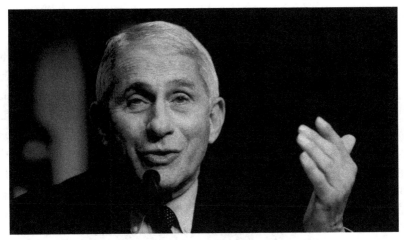

Dr. Anthony S. Fauci, America's Big Brother.

Decades before, during Fauci's long reign over US funded research in the AIDS epidemic, I watched firsthand, in my role as a prominent AIDS and FDA reform activist, the suffering Fauci caused and aggravated by invariably backing FDA delays on approving desperately needed new HIV medications. FDA's risk averse mentality ignores the collateral damage to patients from delays in access to life saving medicines incurred through FDA precautions, particularly in testing the efficacy of new drugs. Impugning treatment alternatives to the Covid 19 vaccines and disregarding the collateral damage to society from the risk hysteria that the FDA habitually induces, has made FDA the foremost DTLM devil behind the details of the draconic Covid policies promoted by Dr. Fauci, FDA, CDC, and many gullible but ambitious blue state governors.

On Covid policy most of the world has blindly followed the US lead and embraced the priorities of FDA and the DTLM as proclaimed by Dr. Fauci. There have been two glaring exceptions, China and Sweden. We have no clear idea of what has really happened or is happening in China, because of heavy handed Chinese Communist Party censorship. China claims only 94,733 cases and 4,636 deaths, that's fewer than Bosnia or Cyprus. Sweden had its own more benign and more sensible counterpart to Fauci, another powerful unelected bureaucrat, Anders Tegnell. In setting Swedish Covid policy, Tegnell ignored Fauci, the US FDA, and our formidable DTLM Complex to follow Swedish common sense.

Mercifully for the Swedes, that country has no exact equivalent of our FDA which left Tegnell free to consider the entire range of Sweden's response options and take into account collateral damage and all of the epidemic's potential tradeoffs. In consultation with other Swedish leaders, Tegnell decided that the damage from lockdowns to their national economy along with the lockdowns painful disruptions of the lives of the Swedish people would likely outweigh the loss of lives that severe lockdowns might prevent. Sweden's Covid death rate was significantly higher than its locked-down Scandinavian neighbors, yet Sweden greatly limited collateral damage by keeping its schools and businesses open while combatting Covid with moderate, flexible measures that minimized disruption of normal life. Social distancing is observed, but masks are strictly optional.

Tegnell's approach saved his country from the destructive social, political, and economic turmoil the Fauci-FDA -DTLM Complex's draconic approach inflicted on the US. However, Sweden was on another planet as far as America's Fauci adoring mainstream media (MSM) and the DTLM were concerned. Fauci and his two most powerful allies, the MSM and the DTLM, rarely gave serious consideration to either the science or the collateral damage from compulsory lockdowns or from the too often symbolic masking before rushing to endorse and make them mandatory.

Fauci, FDA, and the DTLM thought they needed to at least seem to be in charge, to have a plan, and so copied public health procedures from previous pandemics, such as lockdowns and mandatory masking. These had never been tried on a wide scale in a society as vast, complex, diverse and yet interdependent, as America is today. Moreover, we had no evidence that these old methods would work with the novel, highly infectious, Covid 19 virus. Fashioned to deal with the bacterial epidemics of previous centuries, they became a stab in the dark applied to unpredictable, newly emergent, nanoscale viruses. But at least they made Fauci and the DTLM bureaucracies look like they were in charge and doing something useful to stop Covid. Appearances often lie, especially in politics, but they are what counts for the moment, and our MSM always lives in the moment.

A comparison of the State of Michigan (Pop 10.1M), famous or infamous for its Governor Gretchen Whitmer's severe lockdown measures, with unlocked Sweden (Pop. 10.3 M) illustrates the comparative ineffectuality of the Fauci-DTLM endorsed lockdowns. Sweden and Michigan have similar climates and both are industrialized and otherwise highly developed. As I write this, Sweden has had a total of 14,482 deaths among 1,160,465 cases; Michigan has 22,738 deaths among 1,198,850 cases. Public schools in Michigan were closed for months, while those in Sweden remained open without requiring masks. Swedish Covid policies saved vulnerable Swedish children from the terrible consequences of lockdowns, enforced masking, school closures, and social and psychological isolation. Michigan's DTLM lockdown mania inflicted irreparable harm on countless children and their families. Similarly, restaurants and small businesses remained open with minimal losses in Sweden, while in Michigan most were closed, many permanently at the cost of ruined careers and disrupted lives.[4]

US pundits and professional protesters on the left are still giving the DTLM lockdown approach a pass, or even idolizing some of its most culpable leaders. To their great current embarrassment, early in the epidemic they idolized Fauci's now disgraced buddy, quondam TV star and Harvey Weinstein wannabe, ex New York Governor Andrew Cuomo. Criticism of lockdowns and masking comes largely from the right and center right, and that in turn is roundly denounced as "unscientific" by Dr. Fauci and damned for being "pro-Trump" by the mainstream media and kneejerk liberals. It is, therefore, subject to censorship by our tech behemoths, twenty-first century monsters that resemble phantasms sprung from the perfervid imagination of *1984* author George Orwell.

As the legendary Dr. Faustus sold his soul to the Devil to gain magical powers, (the name Fauci, some say, is a diminutive meaning "little Faustus" in the peasant dialect of Calabria) Dr. Anthony Fauci, lacking a soul worth selling, eagerly sold his professional *persona* to the DTLM in exchange for unlimited time in front of the cameras and temporary flashes of political clout. Fauci, as symbol and avatar of the DTLM Complex, remains a folk hero and an infallible scientific authority to legions of benighted Woke ideologues and all those with Trump derangement syndrome, an affliction whose most telling symptom is terminal spite.

Contrariwise, for conservatives and libertarians, this unelected uber-bureaucrat has become a prime villain held responsible for using NIH funding to support the Wuhan lab that appears to have created and released, accidentally or otherwise, Covid 19. They also blame Fauci, not all that unreasonably, for promoting a Covid panic that helped Woke leftists engineer President Trump's election defeat by rationalizing changes in election rules. The changes were done, according to the Democrats, to facilitate voting during a pandemic, and according to Trump supporters to facilitate the left's election cheating. Either way, the changes favored Joe Biden, and they would not have occurred without Covid panic. That made Fauci either a secret savior or an open villain.

Long before handing Fauci the Covid podium, President Trump may have doomed his own re-election bid when, bowing to DTLM pressure, he declined to follow his instincts and appoint reformers to run the FDA. Instead Trump caved to DTLM lobbyists to go with appointees who would refrain from rocking the DTLM's boat. Perhaps following the routine cautions from VP Mike Pence, he also kept Fauci, who in 2017 was 77 and overdue for retirement having ruled NIAID 33 years. For almost as long Fauci had been de facto gate keeper for the entire DTLM Complex encompassing his own NIAID, the NIH, FDA, CDC, and the drug and biotech industries. Under Trump, Fauci's reign over the drug research, development and licensing arm of the Swamp remained as unchallenged as Milton's Satan's reign over hell in *Paradise Lost*. Trump's putting Fauci in charge of combatting Covid 19 was a misstep comparable to Lincoln's initially placing General McClellan in charge of the Union army. Trump, however, never found his Ulysses S. Grant for Covid, and so election defeat ended his chance for replacing Fauci.

Anthony Fauci provides the single most compelling argument for term limits on Federal bureaucrats since the redoubtable J. Edgar Hoover died at the helm of the FBI in 1972. Yet President Biden, who is two years younger than octogenarian Fauci, has assured us there will be no end to Fauci's tenure on his watch. One can see how Biden might feel obligated to keep Fauci whose handling of Covid was a factor, some say the decisive factor, in putting Biden in the White House. Paying political debts, however, seldom insures the best appointees, more often just the opposite. But politics is politics, and so, it seems, we may have to wait for the Spirit Mephistopheles to carry our modern incarnation of the archetypal Dr. Faustus to the warmth of their Satanic master's eternal abode.

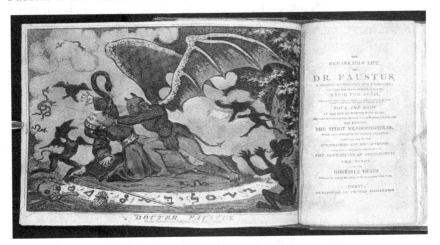

Dr. Faustus meets his end in an earlier incarnation.

Irony of ironies, after inveighing against the DC Swamp for years, when facing the make or break crisis of his presidency Donald Trump turned to the superstar of all Swamp creatures, the physically diminutive but politically formidable Anthony S. Fauci. As the controversy begins to settle from Trump's remarkable presidency, it should become apparent that despite his signal political talents, foreign successes, roaring economy, and domestic policy achievements, Trump's fatal flaw was an ego inflation common to all politicians. In Trump's case ego translated into a flippant initial optimism about the Covid 19 crisis that offended many, empowered his critics, and often made it difficult for him to find and secure loyal, effective supporting talent. Instead, Trump kept on people who had already undermined him, like Dr. Fauci and FDA's duplicitous Stephen Hahn, even as he retained the political double agents running his DOJ and FBI. When it came to appointments, Trump relied heavily on his in house Swamp Creature, VP Mike Pence who turned out to be Paul Ryan in MAGA drag. Too often the results proved ruinous.

Inflation begets recklessness, or *ate*, which in Trump was evident not only in his tweet storms and uninhibited rally rhetoric but in a fatal readiness to trust those who failed to merit his trust. The breaches of trust were many, shocking, and often crippling: most spectacularly with his pusillanimous Attorney General Jeff Sessions, both his openly treacherous FBI chiefs and his first Secretary of State Rex Tillerson. Likewise, his first defense chief General James "Mad-dog" Mattis, and his first Chief of Staff John Kelly quickly turned against him profiting thereby in book sales and speeches, as did National Security Advisor John Bolton and other lesser lights. In his final days Trump was undermined and betrayed by his last AG, William Barr, and gratuitously sold out by Secretary of Education Betsy Devos, whom Trump had loyally supported in the face of sharp criticism. The coup de grace came in a double back-stabbing by that Macbeth-like pair of ice-blooded opportunists, Senate Republican leader McConnell and his Dragon Lady wife, Transportation Secretary Elaine Chow.

But the unkindest cut of all came from the hand of his erstwhile indefatigable yes man, VP Mike Pence, who said "no dice" to Trump at the one moment when Trump desperately needed Pence's loyal support. Had Pence backed Trump on the electoral college challenges, it would have forced Congress and the Supreme Court to do their jobs and give the disputed election the judicial reviews that the gravity of the issue merited, and that Trump's 75 million voters demanded and the American people deserved.

Trump's case for challenging the electors was based on the US Constitution's assignment of control of elections to state legislatures. Democrat governors and state attorney generals used Covid as an excuse to bypass their legislatures in Pennsylvania, Michigan, Nevada, Wisconsin, and other states in order to change election rules. Their changes greatly expanded absentee balloting and loosened restrictions on voter identification, ballot harvesting, vote by mail, and other practices that made cheating easy and enforcement difficult to impossible. There were also widespread issues around voting machine integrity and ballot box security.

In the judgment of various officials, such as Trump's own attorney general William Barr, the cheating was not of sufficient magnitude to affect the outcome of the election. But neither Barr nor anyone else had formally investigated the magnitude of the cheating; besides, Barr lacked authority to rule on the question. His was just another gratuitous Swamp opinion.

It seemed obvious to Trump and his supporters that the Democrats had the will to cheat, and the Covid crisis allowed them to construct the means: the result was inevitable. Congress's constitutional duty was to authorize the election results and Mike Pence's duty, as Vice President, was to accept or reject the legitimacy of contested electors. The Supreme Court's job was to rule on the constitutionality of election changes done by fait by Democrat state governors and attorney generals, as in Pennsylvania, who deliberately bypassed their legislatures. Had Pence done his job, then Congress and the Supreme Court might have been compelled to proceed as the Constitution directs.

Pence's refusal to act on the contested state electors left Americans with the demoralizing lesson that election cheating is all OK as long as it doesn't turn out to be the sole reason you won—which of course we can never know without first identifying the cheating and accurately measuring its full extent. In defense of his refusal to act, Pence raised the preposterous objection that he did not have the constitutional right to perform a task the Constitution specifically assigned to him as Vice-President, the task of evaluating and accepting or rejecting contested Presidential electors. Thomas Jefferson set the precedent by doing just that when he was Vice President. Mike Pence, of course, is no Thomas Jefferson.

Disregarding the Constitution and the rights of the American people to a fair and honest election, and flushing down all loyalty to Donald Trump, Mike Pence instead listened to the DTLM Complex, Silicon Valley, and Wall Street. In an ominous chorus they all were darkly murmuring that any election review would spark months of violent BLM and Antifa riots across the land, very bad for business and the stock market—and a real killer of contributions to future Mike Pence campaigns! As he always had, Pence listened with rapt attention when money talked. Within the LGBT community some murmured that Trump got his just deserts for choosing Pence as his VP. I won't say they are wrong. I will say only that the tens of millions of American people who voted in good faith for President Trump deserved an election with an accurate count of the votes of legitimate, registered voters. Because Mike Pence refused to do his duty, they did not get one and never will. If the intrepid Phyllis Schlafly were alive today, I suspect she would dare to find a more puissant word for Mike Pence's betrayal.

****

Since Dr. Fauci came with the drapes and the carpets, replete with heavy wear, fade, and suspicious stains, trustworthiness was not necessarily expected of him. Still, Fauci and the DTLM's handling of the Covid epidemic, with the overblown risk hysteria they generated and their advocacy of draconic lockdowns, may prove to be the straw that broke the back of Trump's presidency. Although Trump promised to bring the best scientific minds to bear on the pandemic, he didn't bother to find out who they might be or whether they would prove politically trustworthy. Instead, he turned to the bureaucrat "scientists" led by Dr. Fauci, all of them wily Swamp politicians first and scientists second, if at all. Thereby, Trump handed Fauci and his most diehard cronies, the ossified careerists at FDA, a megaphone and a podium that they garrison to this day. As I finish this work in late August 2021, Fauci is getting more daily press than Trump himself. Had Trump thoroughly vetted Tony Fauci politically and professionally, he would have discovered that Fauci is the very personification of the Swamp that Trump repeatedly denounced, and with good reason feared.

Only months later did Trump get around to consulting on Covid with the Hoover Institute's Dr. Scott Atlas in whom he finally found an articulate and willing ally with credible scientific bona fides. By then it was too late: Fauci, FDA, the Pravda media, and their Democrat colluders were dug in. Moreover, Atlas was neither the only or the best credentialed ally Trump could have found, except he never looked very hard or far. Evidently, he or his White House staff didn't want to be bothered.

Like the media buffoons who relentlessly vilified him, Trump appeared to initially trust the government scientists as if they were Science itself. Apparently, he did not realize that by going first to Fauci and the FDA, he, as President, would severely limit his options, empower his political and media opposition, and grant covert adversaries a de facto veto over his Presidential decision making powers on Covid. He would not get them back except by firing Fauci, FDA Commissioner Stephen Hahn, and their lieutenants at unacceptable political cost. Trump has yet to publicly acknowledge that keeping Fauci proved to be an infernal bargain of Faustian proportions.[5]

The folly and tragedy of putting a vain, capricious, and many suspect corrupt, octogenarian bureaucrat in charge of US Covid policies is astounding. Historian Barbara Tuchman could have found in our Covid chaos a powerful sequel to her *March of Folly* review of history's most destructive failures of leadership, over-weening hubris, and delusion in government policy. No well-informed person working in healthcare assumes America's best medical and scientific minds labor as government bureaucrats. Our best are engaged in their own research in beyond the beltway places like Stanford, Yale, Johns Hopkins, Duke, Harvard, Rockefeller University, the Cleveland and Mayo Clinics, or for the biotech or drug companies. Trump should have convened a panel of experts very carefully selected from such places.

At least one of them would likely have advised him, the way Einstein advised FDR to develop the A bomb to insure victory, that the US must undertake an urgent, concerted effort to examine all previously approved and safety tested drugs and supplements to find any that have efficacy in preventing or treating the Covid virus. Drug companies maintain large catalogues of drugs that they routinely test against new pathogens. Trump should have used his panel to put the country on a war footing. He needed their help to launch a highest priority effort to get the entire pharmaceutical industry to identify and test viable Covid treatments simultaneous with his remarkable vaccination effort, Operation Warp Speed, and in concert with his bold efforts to accelerate development of monoclonal antibodies like Regeneron.

Warp Speed was a Manhattan Project for vaccines. However, we needed one for treatments and preventions as well because of vaccine breakthroughs and declines in vaccine efficacy, not to mention those millions who either do not or will not get vaccinated. The people in charge of the treatment initiative needed to be persons without conflicts of interests that disposed them to favor profitable drugs protected under the patents of pharma giants over cheap off patent drugs which would not enrich anyone in the DTLM Complex.

In other words, Trump needed a team whose loyalty to the American people and to humanity itself trumped their loyalty and financial ties to the DTLM. Moreover, the team leaders needed be able to report directly to the President, without having to filter through DTLM potentates Fauci and Hahn. Trump himself understood and stressed the importance of treatment. For example, he brought us convalescent plasma, and pushed through emergency use authorization of Regeneron. However, he had to fight the FDA and the DTLM people in his Administration, and of course they sabotaged his efforts on hydroxychloroquine and undercut him on ivermectin. As of this writing, Regeneron remains underutilized in some areas and has yet to receive full approval from the Biden FDA, although Japan approved it on July 20/2021.

Like millennial students, Trump's own White House staff was not always big on doing homework, and they often had been lax in the exceptionally complex yet essential area of healthcare. Unlike their Democrat opposition, they did not bother to develop a deep bench of politically trustworthy outside healthcare advisors. From such a group Trump needed to recruit people with clout, preferably scientific clout but also political savvy, to set above Fauci and the FDA lifers as a buffer between them and the President. But since such a bench was never developed, Trump had to turn to the political bench he had.

So who did he name to lead the Covid task force? None other than Mike Pence, the Swamp's most predictable yes man. Pence had zero clout visa vis Fauci and the FDA, and he stood gaping in awe of the boundless wealth and lobbying firepower of the corporate DTLM. As Vice President he had devoted what little other clout he had to pressing for administrative infringements of LGBT rights. And that will surely be his graceless legacy! Into the vacuum created by Pence's intellectual and moral fatuity, moved the DTLM's cagiest operator, Tony Fauci, who turned out to be the deadliest of the vipers nesting in Donald Trump's Presidential garden.

Trust the Science, crooned the media buffoons, along with nearly all the Democrats and all too many gullible Republicans. Except with Covid there was no settled science to trust. Science is a complicated process for finding hypotheses that have empirically based *probability*. Empirical science never gives final or certain truths, certainty is the province of mathematics, logic, and revealed dogma. But to tell from the mainstream media and its political fellow travelers, whatever spews from the oracular mouth of the august Dr. Anthony S. Fauci is the scientific equivalent of revealed dogma, shift and flip as it may with the weather or his dentures. To them Fauci speaking on science is, like the Pope proclaiming faith and morals, a font of infallible truth. Science or not, Anthony S. Fauci has joined J. Edgar Hoover as one of the two most consequential and enduring bureaucratic politicians ever to reign over a vast, murky expanse of the DC Swamp. Indeed, Fauci has become the "irreplaceable" J. Edgar Hoover of our healthcare bureaucracy.

Fauci got the initial big boost that propelled him to his Hoover sized prestige and power within the DTLM not from demonstrating any exceptional prowess in science but through a lightning bolt hit of sheer luck during the 1988 Presidential debate. George H. W. Bush and Michael Dukakis were asked to name some of their heroes. Dukakis responded lamely, citing service professions, like teachers and firemen, without naming any specific individuals. Bush boldly named Dr. Fauci:

> *I think of Dr. Fauci. Probably never heard of him. You did, Ann heard of him. He's a very fine research, top doctor, at the National Institute of Health, working hard doing something about research on this new disease of AIDS.*[6]

During Bush's subsequent Administration, Fauci was getting nowhere with his NIAID AIDS clinical research trials. The AIDS activists had been furious with him for years. Like many whose ego size is big and tall, Tony Fauci's imagination proved short and small. Formed in the image of his grand mentor the FDA, Fauci was a plodder who always followed the book, a safe path but not one that ordinarily leads to breakthroughs in science or anywhere else.[7] Finally, Dr. Dan Hoth had to be brought in to re-organize the trials on a larger scale than Fauci used.[8]

But Bush's mention of Fauci was what stuck in the ever constricted minds of the Swamp bureaucrats and the mainstream media.

Bush won the debate, and with it the Presidency. From that moment on, in the eyes of the media and the Swamp, Anthony Fauci became as untouchable as Rosa Parks. As for his actual scientific prowess or lack thereof, no one but the AIDS patients gave a fig. Fauci was the new President's personal hero! —Something no one else in the entire DTLM could claim. That gave Fauci political preeminence above all the lurking creatures of the black lagoon that is the DTLM. And Fauci knew exactly how to use it—to promote Tony Fauci's name, grab publicity for Tony Fauci, and increase NIAID's funding and with it Tony Fauci's political clout!

It is not surprising that NIAID, NIH, CDC, and above all FDA are highly political, although most Americans and our congenitally clueless mainstream media swallow whole the DTLM propaganda that Science alone rules their decisions. Whenever billions of tax payer dollars are involved, politics inevitably enter any picture. Let me cite an instructive anecdote from my previous work *How AIDS Activists Challenged America*:

> *Because its decisions affect a vast swathe of the economy and the lives of everyone, FDA was, is, and always will be a political body. That point was made to me in a memorable way by Louis Lasagna, a distinguished expert on FDA at Yale University who had developed reform recommendations that became popular in the AIDS community. Lasagna told me that President Nixon once called him for advice on finding a new FDA Commissioner. Lasagna offered Nixon three names, listing the merits of each. He then added, almost as an afterthought, "all three are Democrats, but that won't matter, I suppose." There was a long pause at Nixon's end, then Nixon rejoined, voiced lowered, "You suppose wrong."[9]*

After big tech, the pharmaceutical, biotech, and medical devices industries are the most profitable and powerful in America. Unlike Big Tech, which is free of regulation, the lifeblood of profit for all these industries flows only though FDA's licensing and by grace of FDA's tight regulation of their products and services. FDA is the bazooka armed sentry controlling the pearly gates to their paradise of patent guaranteed profitability. FDA supervises all the clinical trials it requires for drug approval. FDA determines the medical claims that can be made in labeling drugs, biologics, and devices, and FDA closely monitors their manufacture. Most drugs are relatively cheap and easy to manufacture. What allows their makers to charge lofty prices is the monopolies FDA grants them. Moreover, for every researcher who relies on NIH and NIAID funding, success or failure of his/her work, along with the big money, depends on FDA licensing profitable products developed from their research.

FDA's enjoys nearly absolute power over the drug and biotech research, development, and marketing companies because neither Congress nor the President have ever exercised effective oversight on FDA, which they imprudently set up as an all too independent agency. FDA's independence is much greater than that of say the State Department, Treasury, or even Defense, over which the President is Commander in Chief and for whom he sets overall policies. Unlike them, FDA acts as if its "credentialed" authority enjoys divine sanction from the great god Science, and in recent decades via Science's avatar, the peerless Dr. Anthony S. Fauci.

Those who decry the damage from drug licensing delays and from FDA's self-serving demands for cautionary overkill know well the crying need for more effective oversight on and accountability for FDA. Patients denied access to life saving medications that are not yet approved pay a heavy price day in and day out for our deficient oversight on FDA.

Nevertheless, FDA has won over to its trademark consumer protectionist risk hysteria nearly the entire Democrat Party, along with the mainstream media, and of course the enthusiastic DTLM. There are FDA critics among Republicans, for example Newt Gingrich in the past and Senators Ron Johnson and Rand Paul currently, but these critics have never marshaled the political support needed to implement fundamental FDA reforms. That would require a President willing, ready, and able to do battle with FDA, its DTLM Complex allies, and their armies of lawyers and lobbyists. Should the voters give him another chance, Trump must make thorough FDA and DTLM reforms his top healthcare priority. Neither the nation nor Trump could survive a second pandemic mishandled and politically manipulated by FDA, Fauci, and the DTLM the ways they did with the Covid disaster.

FDA holds power over the drug companies, CDC, NIH, NIAID, and even over the redoubtable Dr. Fauci because theirs is the ultimate say on approving the results of NIH and NIAID clinical trials. Fauci learned long ago that he must work hand in glove with and for FDA, never against it. Before George H.W. Bush made him a superstar, Anthony Fauci was a competent, though by no means remarkable let alone innovative, government researcher. His true excellence resided in personal ambitions and skills that were exceptionally well-suited to rising in the federal bureaucracy. In short Tony Fauci proved to be a relentless self-promoter, and a bureaucratic manipulator and empire builder, ne plus ultra.

The key to Fauci's long hegemony over the NIH-NIAID-CDC-FDA Swamp, and now the entire DTLM complex, is his very cozy relationship, marriage some might call it, with the king of these beasts, the FDA. His bureaucratic mentality pre-disposed him toward FDA style consumer protectionism. Like a uxorious husband, Fauci always seems happy to let FDA get its way. Never has he been willing to challenge, let alone embarrass, the agency, not even if doing so would save untold human lives. This became painfully apparent to AIDS activists during the early years of that epidemic when, seeking quicker access to new AIDS drugs, they tried in vain to secure a reliable ally in Tony Fauci. He would dally with them, after all he got his name in the news that way, but always he ended endorsing the higher wisdom of FDA's dilatory procedures and its kneejerk risk hysteria. Fauci never lost sight of the signal advantages of giving FDA what they want. And what do regulators want? They want delays, because delays give them power.

However, while FDA Commissioners come and go, there have been eleven different FDA Commissioners so far during Fauci's long reign, Fauci himself enjoys a *de facto* life term like Supreme Court justices, except Fauci has outlasted John Marshall, the longest serving Supreme Court justice in US history. As much as he loves the spotlight, Fauci equally loves his pivotal role of gate keeper. That role allows him to place favorites in high stations, and set up roadblocks and land mines along the paths of those who neglect to bend the knee and kiss his ring or some more intimate part. One of Fauci's all-time favorites, Dr. Margaret Hamburg, worked for years as his girl Friday at NIAID. Fauci at his ear, President Obama appointed Hamburg as FDA Commissioner in early 2009, where she played Fauci's viceroy until 2015. Within the broad expanse of the DTLM Swamp, where Tony Fauci remains the most powerful and enduring tetrarch, the rule for advancement and even survival is, "always suck up to Tony Fauci, opposing him is suicide."

Anthony Fauci happens to be the highest paid Federal employee. According to *Forbes Magazine,* his pay at $417,000/annum is $17,000 higher than the President's, much higher than the Supreme Court Justices, and twice that of mere Congressmen and Senators who serve at the discretion of fickle, easily manipulated voters.[10] Fauci's unparalleled remuneration includes use of the huge mansion provided free to NIAID directors, a benefit offered to neither the Justices nor to Senators and Congressmen. Mitch McConnell's Capitol Hill townhouse is dwarfed by Tony's sprawling abode, as is even Speaker Pelosi's Pacific Heights Palazzo atop her breezy crest in the city by the bay.

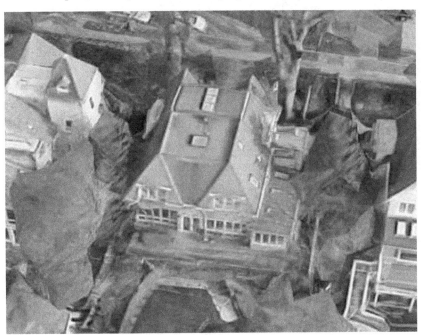

Anthony Fauci's NIAID Provided Mansion

If that weren't enough, Tony Fauci receives many other lush perquisites, like serving on powerful boards topped by that of the richest foundation on Earth, the Bill and Melinda Gates Foundation. Robert Kennedy Jr., one of Fauci's rare liberal critics, has claimed that Fauci may profit through ownership of an element in the Moderna vaccine patent.[11] The charge has been denied but neither disproven nor withdrawn. It seems unsurprising given all the other suspiciously rich remunerations paid to a guy who spends most of his waking hours gabbing with reporters and advising his pals at Google, Twitter, and Facebook on what the American people should or should not be allowed to say, hear, and think.

"Byzantine" a term commonly applied to opaque, ossified, corrupt bureaucracies, is the operative adjective for Fauci's peculiar realm of arcane, daedal medical research. Those able to navigate the DTLM's Byzantine labyrinth stand to gain enviable wealth and lofty professional status, while career death, often with the sudden sting of a stiletto driven Calabrian style deep into the backside, awaits those who fail. Within the DTLM complex the stakes in securing or losing Anthony Fauci's favor can be as ginormous as Fauci's own ego.

In my 1990's role of AIDS activist leader and chief thorn in the side of FDA, I judged him an unscrupulous, self-serving, grandstander as I repeatedly saw how he rewarded shameless shills, marginalized unselfish actors, and repudiated all independent thinkers. Let me relay an incident that says a lot about how Tony Fauci operates. Years later when the PEPFAR and Global Fund International AIDS programs were set up, Fauci, his Bush family connections still intact, rushed to position himself as the gatekeeper and kingpin over these lush new funding streams. Michael Weinstein, CEO of AIDS Healthcare Foundation, the largest AIDS care provider in the US, and I met with Fauci and his top capo Mark Dybull, who was soon to become US Global AIDS Coordinator. AHF had developed the capacity to rapidly set up and deliver high quality AIDS treatment at a reasonable cost. Weinstein sought to offer AHF's expertise and services, wherever they might be needed, to fight the burgeoning global HIV epidemic.

From the outset, it was a bizarre meeting. Fauci and Dybull remained dour and grim faced throughout, as if both were afflicted with severe constipation. When we'd raise an opportunity, challenge, or concern, Fauci would invariably reply with a dismissive wave of his hand, and "we've handled that," or "we're taking care of it," or "it's under control" or "in process right now" or "we're on top of it" or "got the plans all drawn up," or "found the right man for it" or "up and running already," or "all but done." Each time Dybull would nod portentously as if to say, "forget it, you bums!" Fauci had such a plethora of synonymous phrases for giving us the brush off we wondered if he'd cribbed Roget's Thesaurus to prep for our meeting.

AHF got zero support from Fauci, Dybull, or anyone in their sphere of influence. However, the new AIDS money was apportioned to the recipient countries, most of whom wanted to get their people in treatment ASAP. Many chose AHF which, doubtless to Fauci and Dybull's rue, became the largest HIV care provider in the world. Currently, AHF treats more than one million patients in forty-three countries. AHF's success is one of those rare instances where the quality of the services prevailed over Fauci sanctioned bureaucratic antipathy.

This was by no means Fauci's first exercise in selecting who among the AIDS activists he would cultivate and who he would marginalize. Fauci always followed one unbending rule: *give access to and promote only those who support you, and who will never publicly criticize you; marginalize all doubters and potential critics.* That rule works well to insure survival and enhance power in any bureaucracy. Though Tony Fauci's scientific talents may be mediocre, his bureaucratic craft is state of the art.

Fauci, like his all times best buddie the FDA, had his share of conflicts with the AIDS activists over delays in AIDS drug trials and FDA drug approvals. Sometimes these provoked demonstrations against researchers and even incited former screen writer Larry Kramer, the most famous, excitable, and vociferous of the AIDS activists, to call Fauci a murderer. Perhaps not such an exaggeration when we consider how Fauci backed FDA in stalling approval of the drug aerosolized pentamadine to treat pneumocystis carinii pneumonia, while 17,000 AIDS patients died of that terrifying disease during the FDA's two-year delay. Fauci refused the activists request to issue guidelines in lieu of trials, so the patients and their doctors had to set up and run the pentamadine trials on their own. Investigative journalist Bruce Nussbaum relates of the efforts by AIDS patient Michael Callan:

> *Had Fauci two years ago agreed to issue guidelines for doctors just advising them that aerosolized pentamadine might be a good prophylaxis for the number one killer for people with AIDS, nearly 17,000 people might have lived longer. That thought made Callan **very tired**.*[12]

A more common reaction was to make AIDS patients very angry, but Callan's tiredness is understandable since these mortal delays were par for the course dealing with FDA and Tony Fauci.[13]

Fauci would repeat his often lethal practice of backing an ultra-cautious FDA's holdups on approvals and their denials of emergency access to other useful AIDS drugs besides pentamadine, particularly with the antiviral drug ddC. Worst of all, in 1995 Fauci refused to lift a finger to help the activists pressure FDA to give accelerated approval to the protease based cocktails that would turn AIDS from a death sentence to a manageable condition. Had the activists failed in their campaign to move a seemingly immovable FDA, tens of thousands of AIDS patients, denied the drugs that could have saved them, would have died needlessly--more on this crucial juncture in a moment.

Activist Godfather Larry Kramer observed of Fauci:

> *The main reason that Fauci has gotten away with so much is that he's attractive, and handsome, and dapper and is extremely well spoken, and he never answers your questions!*[14]

Not everyone found the gnome-like Fauci "attractive, and handsome and dapper." Michael Weinstein and I did not; "repellent" might be a more accurate term. Yet all the activists feared, if not always respected, Tony Fauci. For his part, Fauci viewed the activists as influential members of a potentially formidable community, some of whom could be induced to become his shills defending him from criticism in the media and helping him by lobbying or running interference for him with Congress. So he sniffed out activists who were ready to brownnose, keeping them close with open access and valuable favors. It wasn't hard for Fauci to recruit eager familiars: at his nod the doors to drug company, NGO, and foundation largess opened like Sesame. Besides, in that time many gay men, so often used to being shunned or marginalized, were eager for acceptance, whatever the strings attached.

Chief among Fauci's gay activist compadres was Martin E. (Marty) Delaney, a former advertising professional who shared Tony's passion for self-promotion. Marty headed the influential San Francisco based Project Inform and gained fame for his advocacy of underground drugs. In 1990 FDA, backed by Fauci, sought to delay approval of the experimental AIDS drug, ddC, in order to run more extensive, and largely pointless, efficacy trials. Fauci liked this delay, since it would require that his very own NIAID run additional clinical trials. Nevertheless, demand in the community for alternatives to AZT, the only AIDS drug FDA had approved, was intense and rising because AZT often had intolerable side effects making its efficacy short lived.

FDA contrived a covert deal with Delaney whereby the agency would look the other way while Delaney's close friend and colleague, Jim Corti, relieved community pressure on FDA to approve ddC by selling an illegal underground knockoff of the drug to the hapless patients.[15] Fauci must have known about and acquiesced to Delaney and FDA's illicit deal and may well have brokered it. He and Delaney always worked closely. I led the community opposition to their medically dangerous, illegal, and clearly immoral scheme, and I facilitated press exposure of the tawdry collusion behind it. For several years Delaney and I remained fiercely at odds over the ddC underground.

When the AIDS drug cocktails that would save millions of lives became ready for FDA accelerated approval in 1995, the stakes rose dramatically. Marty begged friend Tony to help him pressure FDA to award the cocktails accelerated approval. No surprise to me, Marty's entreaties fell on deaf ears. In desperation, Marty turned to his worst adversary in activism, myself. To the gratified amazement of the AIDS patient community, Delaney and I joined forces to lead the drive to compel the FDA to approve the cocktails on an accelerated basis. In that crucial moment, to Delaney's great personal credit, he put the lives of our friends above his animosity toward me and above his extremely advantageous and ever so convenient relationship with the FDA and with Tony Fauci.

FDA needed to provide a rationale and create the illusion of community support for requiring additional trials before approving the cocktails. Fully appreciating the political and financial advantages of their alliance with FDA, the agency's New York based AIDS community shills dutifully launched a raucous campaign, in the press and with public meetings, demanding large simple trials that would delay by at least three years approval for and widespread access to the cocktails. Delaney told me that Fauci privately referred to these shameless FDA shills as "FDA's useful idiots." AIDS patient activists, however, called them different names, like rats and quislings. FDA Commissioner David Kessler laid out FDA's and its shills' joint strategy and rationale in a lengthy lead article in the March 1995 *Scientific American.* To counter Kessler, Delaney, our activist allies, and I persuaded nearly every noted HIV researcher in the country to oppose publicly FDA's and its shills potentially murderous plan.[16]

There was, however, a very powerful hold out, Dr. Anthony S. Fauci. Despite the pleadings from the nation's top AIDS researchers, including Time Man of the Year for 1996 Dr. David Ho, his closest activist friend Marty Delaney, and AIDS patient activists across the nation, Tony Fauci stood by his all-important, career long ally, his ace in the hole, the US Food and Drug Administration. Fauci coveted Ho's honor which might have gone to him had he been willing to show moral leadership by differing publicly with the FDA. Despite the unprecedented stakes in human lives, Fauci declined to support early approval for the cocktails, until of course the deal was done, then he was all for it!

Fauci's strategy was smart bureaucratic politics, and at the same time baldly unethical, par for the course in the DC Swamp. It should have completely discredited him with the activists, but Delaney stepped in to save Fauci's bacon. Not everyone would have done that, but Delaney doubtless saw its value as a chit to be stored up for future use. The FDA's unwarranted delays, which were always to flex their efficacy testing muscle and defend turf, would have cost tens or possibly hundreds of thousands of lives. Turning his back on the activists to implicitly support FDA's deadly delays, Fauci blew his last chance to become a real AIDS hero. Yet no seasoned activist was surprised by Fauci's holding back. We had been dealing with him long enough to know that the only two things in life Tony Fauci would ever risk sticking his neck out for were his alliance with FDA and his own inflated reputation.

Tony Fauci was and remains a true master of cagey, recherché bureaucratic manipulation, like Stalin only with a disarming Italian smile displacing that ominous, black Georgian moustache. Had Fauci a talent for prose, he could have written a worthy modernization of Machiavelli's *The Prince* calling it *The Swamp Overlord.* Anthony Fauci knows the dark recesses of the Washington Swamp the way Niccolo Machiavelli knew the alleys, closets, and bagnios of Renaissance Florence.

One wonders if, in his rare moments of reflection, assuming he has any, Fauci may feel frustration at being born too late for the really big opportunities for power hungry bureaucrats in the Germany and Russia of the 1930s and 1940s, and perhaps born too soon for the truly ominous opportunities that may lie ahead. That early totalitarian era gave us many an example of the dominant qualities the archetypal bad-guy bureaucrat, untrammeled by constitutional restraints, would display. Looking back, we can see how he acts, thinks, feels, and rationalizes his morally problematic actions quietly leading to outright crimes. The quintessential bad bureaucrat would have the "just following orders" ethic of Adolf Eichmann, Joseph Mengele's panache in doing evil, Heinrich Himmler's sangfroid opportunism, Joseph Goebbels ideological fanaticism, Lavrenty Beria's ruthlessness, Stalin's masterful manipulation of everyone and all the rules, and Benito Mussolini's undying love for publicity and self-promotion. Fauci at least has mastered the arts and craft of publicity and self-promotion to a degree that might have incited the envy of Il Duce himself.

According to Bruce Nussbaum, back in the early 1990's a high ranking NIH official called Fauci, "a hit the front page everyday kind of guy."[17] But the Fauci of then was a piker compared to today's media maestro. Marty Delaney, who habitually boasted to grants officers of drug companies about being Fauci's "close personal friend," once told me, "working with him can be rewarding, just remember it is lethal to ever block Tony's path to a camera or mike."[18]

Carl Jung has a term, *puer aeternus* or eternal boy, for the personalities like Fauci, whose moral judgment and sense of social responsibility fails to follow their hair line into maturity. Like a narcissistic boy, Tony Fauci, who will turn 81 on Christmas eve of 2021, always rushes to commandeer center stage. It's almost as if he has to be in front of a camera to assure himself that he's still alive. Fauci appears to have his own variant of Rene Descartes famous cogito where, "I think therefore I am" becomes, "I'm on camera, therefore I must still exist."

Lacking the ego-discipline, exceptional scientific insight, broad-spectrum vision, and imaginative reach needed for making true breakthroughs as a research scientist, Fauci chose instead a more gratifying role as a promoter for plodding, 'by the book' NIH-FDA style "science." Fauci, thus, became a less engaging version of Carl Sagan or a less attractive, pygmy edition of Neil deGrasse Tyson. I always suspected that Fauci was jealous of the AIDS patients and activists back in the 1990's because they, especially the unstoppable Larry Kramer, so often got the role he most coveted for himself, star of the show. After years in waiting as a would-be celebrity, when Covid 19 came along Fauci finally got his big chance for his long coveted starring role, and he went for it like gangbusters — 'step aside Mr. Trump, you're obstructing the camera's view of Dr. Fauci!'

Whenever I saw or met Fauci, I was struck by his adolescent need to appear to be in control, no less than to actually exercise control. The world saw this in his intemperate, borderline bullying, outbursts at Senator Rand Paul in their recent Senate hearing. The appearance of being in control, after all, is crucial to securing a permanent place on center stage. Yet in a combination of Carl Jung's *puer* and shape-shifter archetypes, Fauci's flightiness, evident in his ever-shifting "scientific" opinions, has become the stuff of legends: Masks were useless at first, then required a week later, the next month maybe not needed, and months later you need at least two, and then its three masks maybe clamping them on for another two or three years—need for oxygen be damned. The virus readily penetrates common clothe masks, but we must mandate them anyway, collateral damage be damned. Mandate masks for singles matches in tennis, so what if the players collapse from asphyxiation, CDC rules must be upheld! Mandate masks for children, who except in rare cases neither catch nor transmit Covid, and vaccinate all the kids even if it does give some of the boys life threatening myocarditis. 'Yes, I favor mandatory vaccination; so why the heck is anyone saying I want to force people to get vaccinated?'

Then there's Fauci's infamous, ever shifting story on the origins of the Covid virus told in contradictory bits and pieces under grilling from Sen. Rand Paul. 'The virus came from a bat in a Wuhan fish market, definitely not a lab just a bat. On that lab stuff Rand Paul's a lying dog. He's spreading misinformation about my lab, er' the Chinese lab, and I'll have none of it. But maybe the bat was from some other place in China hundreds of miles from Wuhan, maybe from Mongolia. Well then, maybe partly from a lab. Yes, definitely a lab and probably the one in Wuhan since there's no lab in Mongolia, only bats. But we didn't fund the lab, on that subject Rand Paul's pants are on fire! Except maybe we funded a very minor part of a sub grant to that Wuhan lab. Still, to think again, nature is the virus's most likely origin. There's a whole lot of nature in Mongolia, and its full of bats. I keep an open mind, I'm a scientist after all, so it might be a lab somewhere that was funded to some extent somehow by somebody. But trust me, I resent that bare-faced liar Rand Paul asking me if I funded it. Believe me, he doesn't know a thing he's talking about, and I want to say that officially!'

These Faucian shifts may start out in science but they do not end there. 'It's racist to restrict airplane flights from China,' but six weeks later 'let's ban them from Brazil. Open the schools, no lock them up and throw away the keys. So what if there's zero evidence of significant Covid risk to either students or teachers—we cannot afford to cross the teacher's unions, and they won't budge about school closure. Except all private schools for children of the affluent stay open, mustn't inconvenience any of their bigwig parents.'

Though Fauci's views shift with the political winds, he is consistent on one thing: disagreeing with him on any subject, constitutes disagreeing with Science itself. In his mind, that is a modern, secular equivalent of the sin against the Holy Ghost. "Follow the Science!" "Trust the Science!" blare the slogans from our increasingly Orwellian Pravda media, even though Fauci alters the Science with the weather or more likely with the signals from the Gates Foundation. What doesn't change is the face of "Science," the senescent visage of Big Brother Tony Fauci, the iconic superstar of the trickster-show that passes for federally sanctioned "Covid Science."

Fauci's flip flops along with his wobbly speculations on the source, extent, treatment, and severity of the Covid pandemic characterize Jung's *puer* playing at being a scientist. In addition to his *puer* like shape shifter talents, Fauci displays all the craft of Jung's archetypal trickster positioning himself as the Pied Piper of the cult of draconic Covid 19 lockdowns, replete with sobbing masked toddlers wondering why they're being tortured, masked marathon runners crumpling with CO_2 toxicity, bolted churches, padlocked beaches, barred hiking trails, bankrupt restaurants and hotels in receivership, that swept the world like some hysterical medieval craze, thereby pushing countless small business men and women over the cliff and driving mothers, school children, and college students to despair and even suicide, though not their lucky teachers too well shielded by ironclad tenure and their unions' insurmountable political clout.

So what is "Science" to the media's unhinged group thinkers? — the smiling face of Dr. Anthony Fauci is all that pops up, Big Brother in a white coat! What could be more re-assuring? His "Science" is so easy, even the Pravda media can understand it. "Science" is whatever Dr. Fauci or his DTLM cronies, like Deborah Birx and FDA's Stephen Hahn, said it was in their most recent press conference. Like Newspeak in Orwell's novel *1984*, the meaning of science shifts with the partisan breeze, or with a little badgering from one of George Soros's Woke NGOs, and more recently the on/off spigot of Zuckerbucks. Science is a game staged for the sake and cachet of playing scientist. Forget science as an arduous, meticulous, and never final undertaking to advance our knowledge of nature, that's an anachronism left over from the ancient pre-Covid, pre-Faucian, pre-Zuckerbucks era.

The operative word in Tony Fauci's *puerish* yet nightmarish pantomime of science is "recent." Fauci and his merry media troupe seek to be always on top of things, to be ever the source of the latest "Science."

The reporters from CNN, MSNBC, Bezos Post, and New York Times live in constant need of something new to scurry after, like rats leaping for crumbs from the Pied Piper's lunch. But what if our Covid Pied Piper has no crumbs to drop? In such cases, Fauci re-configures "science" to follow the political drift of the day or the clandestine hand signals from Gates, Google, Bezos, Soros, or Zuckerberg. Thus, to find "science" you must focus on Fauci's most recent pronouncement, whatever it may be. He always tries to give the media something new. Fauci must remain their darling because he lives for press conferences and interviews, indulging in several every day.[18]

For his adoring media, chasing his buzz *du jour* like paparazzi rushing to sneak a snapshot of Justin Bieber or Taylor Swift, Fauci's latest ephemeral pronouncement takes on the glorious cloak of "Science," until his next press conference where the "Science" may well do a mid-air flip. Any who dare voice misgivings about the shifting sands of FauciTruth and FauciFacts may find themselves denied a press card or banned from Facebook, You-Tube, and Twitter, and demoted in search rank on Google and Bing. After all, the public must be protected from purveyors of misinformation, "Science" is sacred, and Tony Fauci is always the latest word on the inside dope of "Science," just ask Fauci himself, he will tell you, "Attacks on me are, quite frankly, attacks on science." The Fauci show must go on, lest people stop, think, question, and doubt![19]

Those who actually practice rigorous experimental science know that, unlike the Fauci *mot du jure*, true science is always provisional, which tends to make real scientists modest. That's something Tony Fauci is never accused of! Science is ever subject to revision with discovery of new facts or by improved understanding of verified empirical data. Although with Fauci it's not the data but the shifting winds of politics that brings the real changes in Faucian "Science." Tony Fauci, as trickster, shape shifter, and *puer,* is the world's greatest virtuoso in applying Bill Clinton's finger to the wind politics to the science of virology! Who would want traditional empirical science anyway? It gives only possibility and probability, never certainty, and politics needs certainty for the moment, whatever moment it may be. You must claim certainty if you want to dupe and manipulate people, mere probability just won't do the trick.

Nevertheless, the nature of science is seldom the reason Tony Fauci is always changing his line or venturing a new speculation based on dubious, incomplete, or invented facts. Like Jung's shifty *puer*, Fauci changes simply to remain the center of attention, to have an excuse for yet another press conference where he can exhibit, play, and promote The Great Doctor Fauci, the incarnate Faustus of our modern pandemic pandemonium. Carl Jung complained that Goethe's Faustus was too often a tiresome windbag. Fortunately for Jung, he did not abide in his mortal coil long enough to have to endure daily briefings from the Faustus archetype's premier 21st century incarnation.

The words of distinguished philosopher of science Karl Popper should be sobering for any still capable of sobriety after listening to the DTLM's Big Brother in a white coat:

> The empirical basis of objective science has nothing "absolute" about it. Science does not rest upon solid bedrock. The bold structure of its theories rises, as it were, above a swamp. It is like a building erected on piles. The piles are driven down from above into the swamp, but not down to any natural or "given" base; and when we cease our attempts to drive our piles into a deeper layer, it is not because we have reached firm ground. We simply stop when we are satisfied that they are firm enough to carry the structure, at least for the time being.[20]

Popper's cautions notwithstanding, NIAID's self-anointed "Voice of Science" stands ever ready to proclaim Science's Verities whenever he feels the urge to hold another press conference. If Tony Fauci has to admit that we have no basis for any new conclusions, novel speculative hypotheses can always be spun upon fragments of data, and every speculation provides an excuse to phone or text a reporter. Fauci talks constantly to reporters and holds repetitious press conferences because that's who he is—not that NIAID doesn't have a public affairs department paid to do those jobs. Instead, NIAID PR is kept busy promoting The Great Dr. Fauci. Of course the Great Fauci makes it easier for them by always managing slightly different angles each time, like "we've got that handled" and "it's under control," and "we're on top of it."

Rarely does the Great Fauci say anything that is new to the scientific community when he Bogarts their mikes. Yet for our besotted media, just by speaking Fauci confers the impressive aegis of "Science" on what from a lesser mouth would be just another 'shot in the dark' conjecture. And so, while Fauci says the same old things repeated in vaguely different ways in slightly varied contexts, the adoring MSM treats his every pronouncement as a ground breaking insight from our uniquely brilliant genius surfacing for a moment from his deep immersion in the "Science." There is, however, a common thread of wisdom in all the varying pronouncements of the Great Oracle of Bethesda: caution, caution, caution, we must wait for and bow to the "Science" which for Fauci means wait for the FDA to delay authentication in order to remind everyone who actually is in charge of sanctioning the "Science," and, most crucial, to delay while FDA and Fauci together decide who they next want to make obscenely rich from their officially sanctioned "Science."

> *But we must not criticize FDA. FDA is infallible, they own the veritable patent on "Science."*
>
> *Just ask the censors at Google, Bing, Twitter, You-Tube or Facebook, or better yet ask President Biden who just asked his High Priest of Science, the legendary Dr. Anthony S. Fauci. "Tony, what's the purpose of FDA?"*
>
> *The Great Fauci replied, "With **a lot** of help from me, and I do mean **A LOT**, FDA decides what is Science and what is not. Then FDA licenses the Science making the licensee rich as King Midas."*
>
> *Patting Fauci on the back, the President chortled, "Tony, I'd like you to have a little chat about FDA with Hunter!"*
>
> *Mr. President, rely on me. I'm definitely your man for that job!!*

Chapter 2

Safe, Effective, but *Unprofitable*

Money plays the largest part in determining the course of history.
— Karl Marx, Communist Manifesto

Covid 19 became the great mass craze of our era, with that sensational team of FDA and Tony Fauci doing what they do best throughout, stoking the fires of risk hysteria, collateral damage be damned. This became shockingly evident with the repurposed drugs hydroxychloroquine, and most important ivermectin, which, used in early disease stage as a drug cocktail including zinc and doxycycline, have repeatedly shown efficacy in quick, small sized clinical studies around the world. For example, some randomized trials indicate that ivermectin used early can reduce Covid hospitalizations and deaths 72%.[20] These drug cocktails are widely, if quietly, prescribed here and across the globe by innovative doctors whose foremost commitment is to their patients. Respected clinicians in the field have stated that by mitigating disease severity these drugs prevented countless hospitalizations saving tens of thousands of lives.[21]

However, FDA is willing to recognize only one form of evidence: that from FDA authorized and supervised randomized double blind placebo controlled trials. Such trials are slow, expensive, and cumbersome to set up in an epidemic where speed of response becomes a life and death matter. Because FDA refused, as it did before with AIDS, to adjust its drug approval standards and pace to the exigencies of an epidemic, most American patients have been denied knowledge of and ready access to Covid treatments that might have mitigated their disease and thereby forestalled many deaths. Possibly, the majority of American Covid deaths might have been avoided with universal availability and standard use of these treatments.

Medical science progressed from witch doctors, shamans, and magic potions to Joseph Lister, William Osler, and Louis Pasteur, and insulin, aspirin, and early antibiotics, all without the help of FDA sanctioned randomized, double blind, placebo controlled trials. Their value is more as an insurance policy against blame for regulatory mistakes, than as a guarantee of safety or a precise prediction of efficacy in individual patients. Human patients are not genetic clones; proof of safety and efficacy in some patients does not guarantee safety and efficacy in all or even in any specific individual. We are learning that yet once more from the plethora of disturbing side effects with the Covid vaccines.

The AIDS epidemic demonstrated, despite dogged resistance from FDA, that where the safety is well established, where we have clinical evidence for basic efficacy, and where the need for a viable treatment is urgent or even desperate, we can save many lives by making experimental drugs available earlier through accelerated approval. Outside of HIV treatments, however, FDA still resists accelerated approval, still resists putting first the needs of dying patients.

The FDA attempted to discredit hydroxychloroquine by instigating some of the agency's most shameless shills, and it has battalions to select from, to raise wildly inflated safety concerns. The drug has been approved for decades for malaria prophylaxis, and used safely, in much larger dosages than for Covid, by millions including this author. Today hundreds of thousands use it regularly for lupus and other conditions.

To discredit the drug, FDA backed one of its special "designed to fail," trials with the wrong dosages administered at the wrong disease stage and without zinc, the therapeutic effect of hydrochloroquine lying in its ability to deliver zinc to cells that need that nutrient to fight Covid. FDA also dug out old safety data on the drug showing some rare heart rhythm issues that would be extremely unlikely to show up in anyone given the low dosage and short duration of the Covid regimen. Then FDA shills rushed to publish, without taking time for peer review, in the esteemed medical journal *Lancet* a scare article which had to be retracted to the embarrassment of that august publication. But not before it had done its damage as blue state governors, with zero medical credentials themselves, stumbled over each other in their spite driven stampede to label hydroxychloroquine "the Trump drug" and issue baseless warnings and crippling restrictions on its use. Why did the *Lancet* publish their attack without the peer reviews that professional standards normally require? We do not know, but experience strongly suggests the hands of a FDA puppeteer pulling strings in the background.[22]

Here in Nevada, where I reside, Democrat Governor Steve Sisolak sprinted to issue intimidating penalties for prescribing and drastic warnings against using "the Trump Drug." The result: conscientious doctors continued to prescribe it early in the disease along with zinc and doxycycline, but only to themselves, their families, and trusted, long-time patients who got Covid. Fearing reprisals from the State of Nevada and the FDA, they held back with the general population, which likely increased the already disproportionately high death rate among impoverished Nevadans and our vulnerable minorities. Governor Sisolak left tolerant Nevadans free to cavort with prostitutes, or blow all their retirement savings at their local casino, or chain smoke reefers to get high as a kite sailing over Caesar's Palace, or use CBD to blur the unceasing boredom of life under his lockdown policies, but God help any caught taking the forbidden "Trump drug" to treat their Covid 19! Such impudent scofflaws faced the implacable wrath of the State of Nevada.

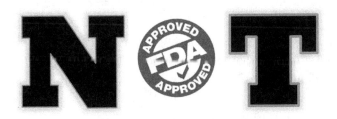

VERBOTEN IN NEVADA!

FDA incites risk hysteria to build its power, increase its funding, and grow its bureaucracy, that's been their *modus operandi* since the thalidomide scare. Thalidomide, which is useful and safe for some therapeutic purposes, had not been tested for safety with pregnant mothers. As a result of this omission, seventeen shockingly deformed babies were born in the US.[23] A far more ominous thalidomide birth was that of the modern FDA itself empowered by the 1962 Kefauver-Harris 'Drug Efficacy Amendment' with a formidable new weapon: interminable efficacy testing rationalized by FDA's trademark risk hysteria.

FDA risk hysteria incites fear and panic by exploiting the human indisposition to wait patiently for balanced risk assessment. When facing a threat, man's hard wired animal impulses are to rush into action, flee into denial, or collapse in fear paralysis. FDA risk hysteria encourages a monomaniacal obsession with a single risk to the exclusion of the wide array of other common risks that confront every mortal human person in his/her daily life. *To manage risks rationally, perspective and proportionality are necessary*. The degree of peril or likelihood of the risk actually transpiring must be painstakingly assessed within the broad context of all the other risks we ordinarily face: the risks of routine accidents like slipping in the bathtub, unforced errors like investing your IRA in Kodak stock instead of Apple in 1997, other diseases like cancer or diabetes, natural disasters like hurricanes and earthquakes, and the ravages of time that come to all.

The entire political and intellectual case for FDA hyper-regulation is built on the agency's covert, and not always so covert but always self-interested, promotion of risk hysteria. It is, of course, highly irresponsible and grossly unethical to whip up risk hysteria simply to further empower or profit one's self or one's employer. Nevertheless, it's par for the course with empire building government bureaucracies seeking to inflate their power and funding. Corporate bureaucracies use similar methods to expand markets and profits: it's their obligation to shareholders, or so they say to evade ethical judgements.

As President Eisenhower warned, the military industrial complex exploits risk hysteria to inflate its budget, numbers in uniform, and armaments, and even to justify launching problematic wars and maintaining obsolete bases and weapons. Likewise, for the entire DTLM Complex, generating risk hysteria is business as usual. The FDA, NIH, and NIAID exaggerate risk to rationalize running more efficacy testing, while established drug companies with products on the market push for ever more efficacy testing as a barrier to entry for new competition.

Few recall, Trump's illustrious Covid Task Force chairman Mike Pence not among them, Jesus's parable of the talents (Matthew 25: 14-30) which warned against risk hysteria, and in effect elevated prudent, rational risk assessment to a moral value. One of this marvelous parable's lessons is that those who selfishly refuse to take risks so that they may realize a greater good lose favor with God and miss out on the best in life. Jesus underscores the risk inherent in living itself, and the crucial need for moral courage in our choices. Shakespeare put it succinctly saying of those who seek life's most ambitious prizes: "Who chooseth me must give and hazard all he hath." The bad stewards in Jesus's parable, like some of the sore losers in Shakespeare's plays, yield to risk hysteria refusing to give and hazard to better their lives or the lives of others.[24]

Tony Fauci may be a little rusty on his Shakespeare and Biblical parables, but he knows that prolonged clinical testing of new drugs is his very own NIAID's bread and butter, the key to holding what he has won and to further empire building. The more feverish the risk hysteria, the more easily Tony can justify protracted, costly, double blinded placebo controlled NIAID supervised clinical testing that will be "needed" to dispel the safety fears that he and his collaborators at FDA are ever ready to generate and fuel.

Fauci's MO recalls popular singer Billy Joel's 1976 hit "New York State of Mind." Billy has many wonderful songs in his repertoire, but Tony seems stuck, like a broken record, humming and crooning out of tune, crackling voiced, renditions of his own not so wonderful theme song, "An FDA State of Mind."

> Some folks like to get away
> Take a holiday from the beltway,
> Hop a flight to dear old Hollywood,
> Or drive down to Atlanta to cavort with CDC.
> But I'm going by Metro to Rockville,
> Taking that old, rattling D Line,
> I'm in an FDA state of mind.
> Let me trip out on FDA risk hysteria,
> Let me blazon baseless fears far and wide online,

Give me FDA's power over riches and human life,
I want to live forever in an FDA state of mind!

Fauci's FDA state of mind manifests an uncontrollable urge to exaggerate and decry any form of health risk in order to delay approval and justify more clinical trials for drugs he or FDA have their own self-interested reasons for delaying. It doesn't matter how remote or minor the risks, how costly the tradeoffs, or how deadly the collateral damage from delay of important treatments. Ask not the reason for the delay, be satisfied that FDA and Dr. Fauci would have it so! Rarely is the purpose of FDA delay to protect the public: control of the markets for drugs is their overriding goal. Only, unlike in Jesus's parable, it is never the selfish stewards, FDA and Dr. Fauci, who pay the price for generating risk hysteria, but rather millions of hapless patients waiting, waiting, waiting, and suffering while they wait some more for better treatments to become FDA approved.

Toni Fauci, with his ever ready FDA risk trigger finger, turns Stanley Kubrick's notorious General Jack Ripper upside down and merges him with Dr. Strangelove. One can easily imagine Fauci adopting for himself one of Strangelove's famous lines: 'today healthcare policy is too important to be left to elected politicians, especially lying fools like that dog Rand Paul!' We saw this in spades with Fauci's endorsing FDA's blatant sabotage of ivermectin and hydroxychloroquine, two unprofitable, off label, off patent Covid 19 treatments with no need for prolonged NIAID safety testing. Yet once more, Fauci was all too eager to lend his crackling octogenarian voice to FDA bureaucrats appropriating decisions that should be left to the citizenry or their elected officials. "Always trust the FDA, it's the Gold Standard!" he'd assure his ever adoring fans in the media.

Within FDA and its allies in the DTLM Complex, any medical risk, however statistically remote, can provide a tried and true excuse for elbowing aside elected officials in order to sabotage common sense healthcare solutions that serve the public interest but run contrary to your specific institutional interests. Serving the public interest is nice, always pay it officious lip service, but never forget that with DTLM bureaucracies, like FDA, CDC, NIH, and Fauci's own NIAID, institutional interest always trumps public interest—and of course that goes in spades for their DTLM corporate allies, and current FDA favorites Pfizer and Moderna are no exceptions.

In this case, the institutional interest that Fauci, FDA, CDC, NIH, the drug companies and their uber-rich front man, medical philanthropist Bill Gates, were chafing to pursue was vaccine development. Indeed, vaccines are the fast beating heart behind Bill Gates' Walter Mitty fantasies of pioneering dramatic medical breakthroughs, and Tony Fauci's little heart habitually beats in tune with big hearted Bill's. They knew there would be huge profits in new vaccines with the US government guaranteeing to promote distribution as well as pay untold billions for them. There would also be career advancement and glory for the researchers, and of course new power for FDA in testing, delaying, and then seizing the hero's mantle to at long last announce the vaccines approval, with multiple cautionary reservations of course to remind us all that FDA is still there "protecting" us.

Tony Fauci, ever entranced in his FDA state of mind, blew several opportunities to become the hero of the AIDS epidemic when he supported FDA's efforts to delay HIV drug approvals in order to conduct more efficacy testing. He may have hoped that by supervising the added testing he could position himself as the hero who saved the world from AIDS. However, the impatient AIDS patients and too many other researchers didn't buy into that plan leaving Fauci high and dry backstage listening to the uproar of applause for Dr. David Ho who was ready to tell the simple truth about the HIV cocktails, they worked!

In the sunset of his life Tony Fauci saw a second chance to become a national hero by snatching the laurels for beating Covid 19 through his role in shepherding development and deployment of Covid vaccines. Forget Donald Trump's essential leadership in launching Operation Warp Speed and bulldozing it through FDA resistance, by definition Trump must be the villain of every Swamp story! At least that's how the Bezos Post, the New York Times, MSNBC, CNN and the rest of our spiteful Pravda media can be relied upon to spin it. And it is their narratives, not the truth, that counts with Fauci, FDA, and the DTLM.

Fauci, FDA, CDC, Bill Gates, the Pharmas and the rest of the DTLM crowd all stood to gain power and prestige by developing Covid 19 vaccines. But even these glorious rewards were overshadowed by the vaccines' humongous future profits. Think of it, a market that potentially could encompass the entire human race! From January 2020 to August 10, 2021 Moderna stock jumped almost twenty-four fold from $20 to $474 raising its market capitalization to $190B, greater than that of Ford, GM, DuPont, and American Airlines combined. And to think, almost no one had ever heard of Moderna twenty months ago! Covid vaccine profits have already minted nine new billionaires, most of them at Moderna and Pfizer, and augmented by 32 billion the wealth of eight existing pharma billionaires.[25]

None of these worthies stood to gain a nickel from repurposed off label treatments of older drugs that have long been safely prescribed, like ivermectin and hydroxychloroquine, let alone from population prophylaxis with cheap vitamin D and zinc supplements. These alternatives needed to be derailed lest they restrict vaccine sales and diminish vaccine profits. And derailed they were by Anthony S. Fauci in league the careerists at FDA, and with bigtime help from their buddies at Google, Twitter, Bing, You-Tube and Facebook. Not to forget, blue state governors, like Steve Sisolak, chafing at the bit to trash any remedy associated, however remotely, with his party's nemesis, Donald J. Trump.

The ever avaricious pharmas were likewise bent on defeating Trump who had the bad habit of keeping his promises to voters. If re-elected, Trump was all but certain to honor his pledge to lower American drug prices down to levels comparable to those paid in other advanced economies. The pharmas are happy to continue to soak American patients disproportionately for their drug research and development costs, thank you! In all his intractable perversity, Donald Trump believed the people who elected him should bear only their fair share of those costs. More of Trump's arrogance in the DTLM Complex's book!

Early in the epidemic the possibilities of alternative ways of combatting Covid through vitamins and nutritive supplements were explored and proposed. In regard to vitamin D prophylaxis, futurist Raul Ilargi Meijer posed a thought provoking query:

"People who get enough vitamin D are at a 52 percent lower risk of dying of COVID-19?" Why have these people died? Vitamin D plays a crucial role in the immune system and may combat inflammation. These features may make it a key player in the body's fight against coronavirus. Rates of vitamin D deficiency are also higher in some of the same groups who have been hardest hit by coronavirus: people of color and elderly people. Why is there not one single country that has a nationwide program to boost vitamin D levels in all its citizens when both death and infection itself could be lowered by some 50%?[26]

The case for social distancing as prevention has been well confirmed. The case for large scale vitamin D prophylaxis cutting Covid deaths and hospitalizations remains largely unconfirmed because it hasn't been tried in any controlled environment. Vitamins cannot be patented, so no private company could afford to run a trial of Vitamin D as prophylaxis. NIH could do so, but it only runs trials in conjunction with drug companies and the FDA. Why is that? —well, ask them and ask your Congressperson.

FDA has for decades wanted to drive the vitamin and supplements industry out of business by over-regulating them into bankruptcy. Doctors learned in the 1980s that folic acid, otherwise known as vitamin B9, given to mothers early in their pregnancy could prevent *spina bifida*, a fatal birth defect. For more than twenty years FDA pursued various legal maneuvers to prevent folic acid manufacturers from advertising this benefit. FDA maintained that the manufacturers were using folic acid as a drug, and therefore it was subject to FDA regulation. (If FDA thought they might get away with arguing that water is used as a drug to treat thirst, they would attempt to regulate your local water department!) Mary Ruwart observes:

Had the US folic acid manufacturers been permitted to advertise the benefits of their product back in the 1980s, . . . we might have seen a decline in birth defects. Instead, more than 10,000 babies were born with deformities more horrible than those with thalidomide. Thousands more were aborted.[27]

Vitamin D prophylaxis for Covid 19, like folic acid for *spina bifida*, was a non-starter, not because it was a bad idea, but because it was an FDA blocked idea that ran contrary to the interests of the DTLM Complex.

The cases for prevention by mandating selective lockdowns, school closings, and those sieve like cloth and paper masks in common use are at best problematic, yet there have been curiously few rigorous attempts to confirm their value with further studies. Is this because the authorities know that rigorous randomized control studies would only show that these steps are mostly symbolic and therefore would weaken the cases for mandatory masking etc? The recent release of Fauci's emails reveal that he sensibly believed, though he would never state it publicly, that the miniscule Covid 19 viral particles can slip right through masks other than the M95 level masks. The evidence we have indicates that Fauci got this point right.

Yet health departments across the world continue to mandate masks, even for those exercising outdoors where there is no significant Covid risk and the masks clearly create serious breathing impediments that outweigh the value of the minimal protection they might afford against a close to non-existent threat. The most fundamental rule of medicine is "First do not harm." Why do health departments disregard that rule when it comes to their mandatory masking? They also continue to mandate job extinguishing lockdowns in many low risk work situations they deem "non-essential" without explanation. With little or no scientific justification, they mandate demoralizing school, church, sports, and restaurant closures. However, as Meijer points out, not a single country has officially suggested that their populace try treating its Vitamin D deficiencies. All those derelict public health bureaucrats across the globe must be crooning with Tony Fauci his broken record theme song, "An FDA State of Mind." For want of thoughtful health policies, they just "sing along with Tony."

Here and elsewhere, FDA's trusty Tontos, Google, Facebook, Twitter, You-Tube, and Bing, have kept busy running interference for the agency by stacking search results in favor of FDA's "authoritative" positions, banning discussion of verboten yet safe and probably effective Covid drug cocktails based on hydroxychloroquine or ivermectin, and through de-platforming their advocates. Of course they must protect the public against false information! What better way than by making sure that your searches can access only "authoritative truth" according to our glorious FDA and 'America's Official Science Genius,' our DTLM Dear Leader and Big Brother, Dr. Anthony S. Fauci? FDA is after all the "gold standard" for drug and device evaluation and information. As for Dr. Fauci, the tech giants swear on a stack of Communist Manifestos that He is infallible in all matters of Science and Medicine!

Follow the money! Treatments like vitamin D, Zinc, ivermectin, and hydroxychloroquine are off patent and dirt cheap. Tens of millions already take them for other conditions so we know their side effects too well to justify further safety testing by Fauci's shop. DTLM insiders professed concerns that these off label treatments might undercut support and the rationale for enormous public outlays to develop and deploy their vaccines. Fauci and others referred to a federal rule that vaccines should not be given emergency development if there are existing, approved treatments. But this is real life, not a fairy tale where arbitrary, unalterable dictums from some shadowy father figure set the narrative. Such concerns were unwarranted because Congress and President Trump were ready to spend "whatever it takes" or make the rule changes required to develop a Covid 19 vaccine. Whatever is Congress for but to change laws that need to be changed?[28]

FDA and Fauci knew this of course, but they wanted to make sure their vaccines had no competition from any inexpensive, off label, off patent treatments. To crush the alternatives, FDA did what it habitually does, instigate risk hysteria. Indeed, using scare tactics is a kneejerk reaction for them. The existing off patent treatments might have saved lives, but at the wholly unacceptable cost of reduced vaccine profits, and even worse it could have sidelined the FDA and Tony Fauci! Take away Tony's mike and the cameras, and his ego would begin to shrink and dissolve like a drenched Wicked Witch of the West. What a tragic sight!

Still, a little imaginative leadership on the part of the Trump White House might have made a big difference had it been tried. It would have cost comparatively little to launch a campaign to inform the public of the mitigation benefits of taking vitamin D and zinc; swallowing a pill is a much lesser nuisance than mandatory masking. Our government could and should have urged doctors to consider prescribing drug cocktails of ivermectin or hydroxychloroquine with zinc and doxycycline *early* in the infection while using Regeneron as a backup for more severe cases of Covid. There was no proof positive that these treatments would work in all patients, but they are safe drugs when prescribed at low dosages so nothing would be lost if they failed. Where the risk is nanoscale, in a free country it should be left to the doctors and their patients to decide whether to take a treatment. Regulators should not be micromanaging family physicians. Some studies have shown that, when prescribed early, these cocktails can lower Covid death rates by up to 72%. But even a 52% lower death rate with easily administered vitamin D supplements would have allowed schools and small businesses to remain open in most circumstances.

Granted these alternatives have not been tested under the "FDA Gold Standard," the agency's plodding, interminable, and wildly expensive randomized double blind placebo controlled trials. But guess what, neither have compulsory masking and mandatory lockdowns been tested that way. Indeed, we lack evidence that could meet strict FDA standards for the safety and/or the efficacy of simple cloth or paper masking used to prevent Covid transmission. If to be sold for Covid protection these simple masks needed to pass strict FDA standards for devices, they'd probably be rejected as ineffective and, yes, unsafe because they restrict breathing and collect viruses, spores, dirt, and colonies of bacteria, all of which are hazardous for humans. More likely, FDA would require M95 masks which are theoretically Covid proof yet very difficult to wear correctly, as well as expensive and in short supply. All masking has serious, seldom mentioned, safety issues, especially with children, athletes, and individuals with breathing or lung problems. It can cause CO_2 toxicity and oxygen deprivation, not to mention the psychological problems from social restriction and isolation. With everyone masked, no one ever gets a smile, and that may be one reason why this country and the world are in such a foul funk. How often have Dr. Fauci, CDC, and FDA warned against these risks? How often have you seen hogs fly?

The simple masks in common use are effective in one political respect: they are a posturing rite designed to give a re-assuring sense of doing something where nothing effective is being done or can be done, at least nothing effective according to strict FDA safety and efficacy standards. However, mandatory masking echoes very dark times in history when compulsory articles of clothing were used to symbolize subservience to the power of the government. They remind us of the yellow stars of David and the pink triangles Jews and gays were compelled to wear in ghettos and Nazi concentration camps. They also recall the various symbolic accoutrements that slaves wore throughout the ages to signify their degraded status.

Masks do keep us occupied so we don't think too much while waiting for FDA's preferred solution, the vaccines. For many people wearing a rosary or a Buddha or Ganesh medallion, or bowing to Mecca might help as much or as little as wearing a mask. In a supposedly free country, that would not justify government mandated rosaries, Buddhas, or prayers to Mecca. At their most innocuous, masks are the grand placebo of the Covid pandemic. But their underlying purpose is less to protect us from Covid than to create the illusion that the government, that is Fauci, FDA, and CDC, knows what it is doing, is in control, and, therefore, must not be questioned but only obeyed.

Covid spreads indoors in confined spaces. All the evidence indicates that, except in intimately close contact, it does not spread outdoors. Masking outdoors to prevent Covid is clearly unnecessary, and unhealthy for persons engaged in physical activities, such as running, that increase the breathing rates. Yet schools, athletic events, and local governments have required outdoor masking. Why have Fauci and CDC not spoken out against unnecessary outdoor masking and issued guidelines warning of its health dangers? Their epidemic management is a fatal mixture of rigid ideology, self-serving diktats, and rank incompetence.

Notwithstanding, we have very good evidence that conscientious social distancing does work, and should be practiced even outdoors. So why not enforce social distancing more rigorously and make masking voluntary? The answer is simple, social distancing lacks the symbolism of masking; you can't wear it, and it doesn't effectively signal your submission to Big Brother.

What is the fundamental reason why simple, safe prophylactic and inexpensive mitigation efforts like vitamin E and ivermectin are never given serious consideration by Fauci, CDC or FDA, while hazardous and often useless masking and always destructive lockdowns are mandated? A major reason, is surely vaccine profits, but an even more fundament reason lies in *the nature of bureaucracy*. Modern states set up special bureaucracies for dealing with problems like Covid 19. It's the job of the fully credentialed "scientific authorities" in the medical bureaucracies, that is FDA, NIH, NIAID, and CDC, to authorize solutions to medical problems. It's not the job of the people's elected representatives, these overlord agencies' affronted bureaucrats will insist, and certainly not the job of thought leaders in extraneous areas—for example, political, religious, or business leaders, or economists, humanists, lawyers, artists, et al---to meddle in medical matters where they lack professional credentials and proper authority. In other words, "get the hell out of DTLM turf!"

By the same type of perverse turf thinking, we should leave it to the Pentagon to decide if, where, when, and how our country sends its youth to die in foreign wars. Instead, Congress is empowered to decide whether or not we will go to war, and to evaluate and criticize the military's conduct thereof. The Constitution requires Congress to issue a declaration of war before the President and the generals can legally launch a war. While Congress may stand up to our Lords of War in the Pentagon and hold them strictly accountable, FDA, CDC, and NIH did not yet exist when the founders wrote the Constitution. Consequently, the Constitution has no provisions specifically tailored for governing and disciplining powerful overlord agencies like the FDA, CDC and NIH let alone for the FBI, IRS, DEA, or CIA.

Nevertheless, these later emerging swamp monsters can be more formidable within their own domains than is the President or the Congress. No wonder the President, Congress, and other elected leaders are afraid to cross the overlords of the three lettered agencies. This has been especially true during Covid, with respect to the DTLM's unofficial Lord of Lords, its Dear Leader, Dr. Anthony S. Fauci, and his High Sparrow, the Commissioner of the FDA.

Consequently, Congress, with a few undaunted exceptions like Senators Rand Paul and Ron Johnson, has largely abdicated oversight on these worthies as well as on rest of our vast array of increasingly autonomous overlord agencies. *The FDA, CDC, NIH, and NIAID, along with the FBI, CIA, DEA, and IRS, are becoming the real powers in our bureaucratic age as their regulations replace or supersede bona fide legislation.* Thus, America is unknowingly slipping into a neo feudalism where the greatest powers of the land are no longer Congress and the President, our equivalents of Parliament and the King, they are instead the unelected feudal barons of the 3 lettered overlord agencies. Omnipotent within their domains, they have their own equivalents of armies and intelligence services, their own vast revenues etc., and are accountable to no one, least of all to the people who must learn the hard way never to cross the overlords. The Constitution made the people sovereign, but their sovereignty has gradually been forfeited, lost piece by piece, to these all powerful overlord agencies and the closed professional guilds that control them.

Intimidated as a group during the Covid pandemic, few of our elected representatives dared speak out against the DTLM bureaucracies' "scientific authorities" usurping Congress's constitutionally delegated responsibility to oversee all aspects of governmental operations, which would include oversight on the FDA-CDC-NIH centered guilds that presume to call themselves "Medical Science." One of the people's representatives who did speak out was Sen. Marco Rubio:

> *The American people deserve the truth, they also deserve accountability. When elected representatives make decisions, they can be held accountable by the public. But when public health officials with decades of experience and leadership within our nation's institutions short circuit the political process and make decisions themselves they deny the American people that same opportunity—and to change course if desired.*[29]

Senator Rubio must have been woefully ignorant of the *FAUCI-FDA-CDC-NIH overlords' royal rule* for dealing with American citizens and their duly elected representatives—*OUR WAY OR THE HIGHWAY!* As Donald Trump discovered to his rue, that rule applies to Presidents even more than to mere Senators and Congressmen, especially to Presidents named Trump. The DTLM rule enjoys fervent backing from the mainstream media, where the DTLM maintains battalions of shills (they deserve a worse name!), and from the tech behemoths eager to curry favor with all government bureaucracies. The DTLM and the tech giants' sage advice for the ignorant hoi polloi, for instance Senators Marco Rubio, Rand Paul, and Ron Johnson, along with their unwashed, benighted constituents, is just to sit back quietly waiting for the judgments of "the experts," that is the anointed bureaucrats led by their revered spokesman-for-life Dr./St. Anthony S. Fauci, backed by his acolytes at NIAID, NIH, CDC, and, most important, sanctioned and authenticated by the Holy of Holies, the US Food and Drug Administration, Savior of the Nation from the Horrors of Thalidomide!

Dr. Fauci and his acolytes, admirers, and co-colluders were no more inclined to mitigate Covid with alternative therapies than they were to listen to impertinent carping from the people's elected representatives. Alternative therapies and inexpensive mitigation are not what the DTLM does, because they are never highly profitable in any way to anyone in the DTLM Complex. Yes, we need ways to curb Covid 19, but you (the American people) will be allowed to use only those ways authorized by the DTLM, ways that protect and expand the DTLM/s turf and its professional privileges and, above all, further its enrichment.

Despite their mono strategy of relying almost exclusively on vaccines (backed by posturing with flimsy clothe masks and arbitrary lockdowns designed to instill obedience in the populace), FDA and the DTLM nonetheless delayed getting their vaccines out. Peter Suderman in *Reason* contends that at strategic junctures the FDA resorted to its tried and true dilatory crafts in order to slow vaccine development and, especially, rollout.[30] He writes:

> *The most glaring example of the FDA slowing down the process was at the very end. After conducting multiple, increasingly large clinical trials throughout the year, as the FDA requires, Pfizer-BioNTech submitted an application for emergency use authorization on November 20. The relevant FDA panel did not meet to approve the request until December 10, which meant the first vaccine was not administered until December 14.*
>
> *The FDA could have met immediately, on an emergency basis, reviewing paperwork and data collection on a rolling basis so*

that by the time the application came in, they were ready to give it the go-ahead. This is not some hypothetical alternative that doesn't work in the real world; it is <u>what drug regulators</u> in the U.K. did last year. . . . If the FDA had been willing and ready to approve the vaccine on the day the application was submitted, the vaccine rollout could have started weeks earlier.

An even more costly mistake, Suderman continues, occurred earlier in the process:

it's possible to determine efficacy much more quickly, via a process known as human challenge trials, in which volunteers are intentionally, exposed to the virus. Human challenge trials provide actionable data much faster and with far fewer subjects than more conventional large-scale trials, making them particularly excellent tools for emergencies . . . . In February, the U.K. approved compensated COVID-19 human challenge trials, . . . These sorts of trials, however, could have been approved here in the United States by the FDA last year, dramatically speeding up the final phase of testing.

Such emergency steps by FDA might have forestalled tens of thousands of American Covid deaths, reduced the staggering damage to the US and world economies, and thereby prevented collateral deaths worldwide from delayed care, poverty etc. Yet FDA stalled vaccine development, testing, and roll out again, as always, in the name of safety. But safety for who? –the patients and the whole of humanity desperate for relief from Covid, or safety for FDA's institutional authority and reputation? FDA made that decision, but in a democracy a decision that impacts the lives of all citizens should be made and finalized only by those properly elected officials who have constitutional oversight upon the FDA and the rest of the Federal bureaucracy. But they, as Senator Rubio protested, were never consulted. It is increasingly evident that oversight on Federal bureaucracies of any stripe is becoming a lost art in contemporary America.

Why would FDA backed by the DTLM complex and Dr. Fauci want to delay the vaccines at the likely cost of human lives? Their most pressing reason was politics. To get the vaccines out before the 2020 election might have insured the re-election of Donald J. Trump. A re-elected President Trump might have listened to Senators Ron Johnson and

Rand Paul, as well as to his backer Peter Thiel and all the conservative thinkers urging him to appoint true reformers to overhaul our sclerotic FDA and dysfunctional CDC. Almost certainly, a re-elected Trump would at least have seen that Tony Fauci got his fool's gold watch and walking papers.

Even more disturbing and utterly unacceptable to the corporate DTLM, a re-elected Trump would have proceeded with his widely popular efforts to curb pharmaceutical price gouging. Although any unnecessary delay in approving the vaccines would cost thousands of lives, FDA could not resist the temptation to delay given the stakes for the agency's powers, for their ever faithful ally Tony Fauci's tender ego, and for DTLM corporate profits.

After all, who could call FDA into account? That agency knew from experience that our system has long failed to provide effective oversight on itself or on any of the similar independent Swamp overlords, especially not on Dr. Fauci's very own NIAID. With effective oversight and strict accountability, the Swamp would no longer be a swamp, and where would the poor displaced Swamp creatures find a place to call home? Without their sinecures, they might actually be forced to find real work. Imagine the humiliation FDA lifers would feel if forced to engage in productive work to pay their mortgages.

Besides FDA's aggressive efforts to block use of existing products and drugs for prophylaxis and treatment of Covid, a third extremely costly DTLM mistake was Fauci's and the CDC's failure to move quickly to identify, isolate, and protect those most vulnerable to the disease. Mainstream media's refusal to call them into account for failing to protect the vulnerable elderly, especially those in nursing homes, further aggravated the total damage. Instead, time and scarce resources were spent on the under the forty population and even on school children who are statistically at less risk of dying from Covid than of accidentally drowning in a swimming pool. Ask not their reasons why, the DTLM's charge is but to profit or die!

Early statistics from Italy revealed that the overwhelming preponderance of deaths and hospitalizations with Covid were in patients over 65, especially those with underlying conditions such as diabetes, respiratory and cardiac diseases, and morbid obesity. The mean age of death with Covid 19 has been over 75, whereas in 1990 the mean age of death with AIDS was under 40. Yet in place of swift actions to protect our vulnerable elders, the FDA, Fauci, the corporate DTLM, and all too many blue state governors backed one size fits all politically motivated lockdowns.

Their lockdowns closed the schools, needlessly inflicting unfathomable hardships on tens of millions of children and their parents along with millions of college students. Restaurants and shops were shuttered, decimating the hospitality industry and other small businesses. Outdoor dining, open air sports and both inside and outside religious services were banned, despite overwhelming evidence that the virus almost never spread outdoors. All the while windowless big box stores were kept open for land office business. In fact, no explanation, scientific or otherwise was offered for keeping large establishments open while closing smaller ones. The big stores were arbitrarily designated "essential services." It was all done by diktat. But, then, who wants to tangle with Walmart, Kruger, Costco, and Target? Not Tony Fauci for sure, he's the little friend of every organization that's monstrously big. One thing was sure, someone needed to suffer to show how seriously we are taking Covid 19, so let it be the small businesses. Their owners vote Republican anyway.

Even the Fox newscasters have generously attributed the closures to Fauci's, the CDC's, and the blue state governors' stupidity and fanaticism. Follow the money and you'll get a more mercenary explanation. By maintaining the fiction that everyone, infants, school kids, college students and healthy people under 40 needs to be vaccinated, the DTLM complex tripled the potential market for their vaccines which still would have been immensely profitable if given only to the vast numbers who actually need them.

Despite Trump's justifiably, if bombastically, decrying the dangers of the DC Swamp, he too often proved helpless in either identifying or remedying the specific problems with the Swamps' bureaucratic response to Covid 19. Before running again, Trump should bone up on Teddy Roosevelt's trust busting and develop ways to apply it to the governmental overlords especially the FDA, NIH, NIAID, and the

FBI and CIA. If he doesn't run again, he can do the nation an immense service by insisting that any candidate he endorses must pledge to fight for effective oversight on the three lettered Swamp overlords, including subjecting them to trust busting measures.

Of course, Trump was handicapped because being President made the federal bureaucracy his unloved and very unloving stepchild. Notwithstanding, he should have exposed the self-serving motives and conflicts of interest behind the DTLM's resistance to utilizing existing treatments. Had he understood better the character defects and malign motives of his adversaries in FDA, CDC, NIAID, NIH, and the rest of the DTLM Complex, he might well still be President.

Donald Trump was far more reasonable, patient, and even kind to them than they ever deserved. The generous streak in his often impulsive nature, something he rarely gets credit for, may have blinded him to their dark motives. The same, of course, might be said of his dealings with the FBI and DOJ at the onset of his presidency. A second major handicap was his magnanimous trust of and reliance on Mike Pence for vetting and supervision of appointments in healthcare. Too often that meant placing politically unreliable people, such as Fauci, Birx, and Hahn in high places where they spitefully undermined Trump with impunity. Not to mention all the Pence people bent on antagonizing the LGBT community whose power in the voting booth and in the general culture too many Republicans underestimate to the GOP's detriment. Unlike Mike Pence, Donald Trump does understand that the GOP cannot afford to permanently cede to the Democrats the 6% of the electorate that self-identifies as LGBT.

Despite resistance from FDA, Trump's bold initiative with Operation Warp Speed appears to have accelerated by at least a year development of viable Covid vaccines—an amazing achievement considering that experts, including the omniscient Fauci, at first said that developing a vaccine for a new pathogen would take at least three years. Trump accelerated FDA's cumbersome processes and eliminated many, though not all, of their delays by applying very heavy presidential pressure on the agency and the rest of the DTLM complex. Moreover, at Trump's behest, the government paid to speed manufacture of the vaccines so they would be ready in tens of millions of doses when approved. To accelerate development further, Trump stipulated that the government would pay the developers for the vaccines even if they did not work! With these bold initiatives, Donald Trump likely saved hundreds of thousands of American lives and prevented far worse devastation of the US and world economies.

Given Trump's political opponents merger at the hip with the DTLM complex led by Tony Fauci, and given the FDA's kneejerk instigation of risk hysteria, had one of theirs controlled the White House in 2020 the epidemic's death toll and its dire economic fallout might well have become truly catastrophic. It still may, due to the mindsets of some of those currently at the helm. Imagine the Federal response under a President Cuomo, Newsome, Pelosi, or Whitmer. As for Joe Biden, he *seems* kinder and gentler than the others, at least if you don't ask American citizens trapped in Afghanistan. But who knows who's really in charge of the Biden White House?

Given the open *animus* toward Trump throughout the MSM, Hollywood, Silicon Valley, and academia, and the covert support from their patron saint, Tony Fauci, we'll see a white out in hell before the DTLM complex and their spite driven allies in the media and academia give Donald Trump one iota of the credit he deserves. But let me, for my part and for the record, give credit where credit is due: **By rushing the Covid vaccines through a recalcitrant FDA at unprecedented speed and by guaranteeing to pay the companies for them regardless of whether they worked, President Donald Trump saved countless American lives and prevented what could have become an economic disaster as severe as the Great Depression. It was Trump's parallel to FDR's quietly preparing a reluctant America for World War II. The very qualities for which Donald Trump is so often harshly condemned, willfulness, impetuosity, and thinking outside the box to over-rule "the experts," probably saved America and the world from unmitigated catastrophe. At least there's hope he saved us, but who knows what damage the crew around Biden will yet do.**

Chapter 3

The DTLM in the Mirror of History

There is a need to draw a line between leaders responsible and the people like me forced to serve as mere instruments in the hands of the leaders. I was not a responsible leader, and as such do not feel myself guilty.
— Adolf Eichmann

Let me pose an intentionally shocking, deliberately loaded question designed to upset apple carts and spur radical re-thinking. *Did the self-serving delays of our Drug Testing, Licensing and Marketing establishment, headed by FDA, NIH-NIAID and their avatar Dr. Anthony S. Fauci, kill more Americans by blocking use of treatment with alternative drug cocktails for Covid 19 than Dr. Josef Mengele killed Jews, gipsies, and gays with his demented experiments using human guinea pigs?* The answer may well be yes, although many will cry foul to the question. Certainly, the personalities, methods of killing, and motives were quite different.

Mengele was a deeply evil Nazi ideologue who manifested the darkest side of Jung's ever cagey trickster archetype. Fauci is a vain, arrogant, yet gelidly calculating Swamp bureaucrat distinguished mainly by his abiding love for self-promotion and near genius knack for getting publicity. But Fauci is also a total ideologue in his commitment to FDA's trademark risk hysteria, to plodding, unimaginative 'by the book' FDA style science, and to big government hyper-regulation. These are reinforced by his refusal or inability to think in terms of drug approval trade-offs, an art that requires honestly weighing the overall risks to individuals and society in delaying valuable treatments against the hazards for the FDA and the DTLM of being proved wrong with a premature approval, as they did disastrously with Vioxx in 2004. Like FDA, Fauci always weighs the risks to the bureaucracy far more heavily than the risks to the citizens the bureaucracy was established to protect and serve. Fauci appears to suffer a mental block preventing him from grasping the concept of collateral damage. Like one of today's fashionable neo-Marxists, Tony Fauci thinks in terms of bureaucratic authority, credentials, regulations, rules, and groups, not in terms of freedom and rights for individuals, let alone justice as applied to individuals.

At Auschwitz Dr. Mengele, the trickster as Nazi ogre, performed diabolical experiments torturing and murdering his victims and even putting human body parts to grotesque, abominable uses. In most layman's eyes the sometimes deadly procedural delays of FDA, self-servingly defended by Dr. Fauci and the entire DTLM complex, would have nothing in common with the Nazi's inhuman experimentation. Notwithstanding, taking a view from the mountain top, both are historically important cases of bureaucratic arrogance motivating destructive scientific experimentation on unwilling human victims.

In Mengele's case the evil acts and their motives were blatant. In the case of Dr. Fauci, the FDA, and the DTLM their bad, self-interested motives are concealed from a somnolent public and an obtuse Congress by a biased, willfully negligent media and a quasi-totalitarian big tech. In many cases their motives are hidden from themselves via group-think denial. As Eichmann might have said, they were only following their organizational rule book; or so they would have us believe and on that basis exonerate them from all blame and any whisper of censure. The fact remains that they impeded, and where feasible they blocked, use of ivermectin and other safe treatments that increasing numbers of reputable doctors around the globe claim can reduce Covid deaths and hospitalizations by up to 70%. They lacked medical or moral justification for interfering with the free choices of doctors and patients, and had no sound legal authority for doing so. Indeed, shutting down public discussion of the treatment alternatives, in a totalitarian spirit, recklessly endangered public health. Worse still, they were motivated by greed: they wanted to increase the markets and profits for their vaccines, and they wanted all the credit for stopping the virus to go to themselves.

Commenting on his July 19/2021 Senate kerfuffle with Dr. Fauci, Sen. Rand Paul pointed out that in 2012 Fauci let slip his deeply problematic motive for colluding with the Wuhan lab on their fateful gain of function research. The benefits from gain of function research, Fauci maintained in words couched in characteristic cageyness, outweighed the risk of that research accidentally triggering a deadly pandemic. To quote Fauci:

> *In an unlikely but conceivable turn of events, what if that scientist becomes infected with the virus, which leads to an outbreak and ultimately triggers a pandemic? . . . I have said – that the benefits of such experiments and the resulting knowledge outweigh the risks.*[31]

We're moved to shout whoa! Who is Tony Fauci to decide that? And what risks to whom? To the researchers, or to the entire human population? Fauci's playing God here. Or, like Dr. Faustus, he is selling his soul for today's scientific equivalent of forbidden black magic.

Here we see the arrogance of the scientist at its worst, blithely assuming that his pursuit of scientific knowledge justifies the taking of human life, and that he personally has a right to make that decision. So Dr. Fauci, in thought at least, commits Dr. Faustus's sin of paying any price for knowledge, and that sin is Dr. Mengele's prime sin as well. Like Faustus in his quest of forbidden knowledge, both Mengele and Fauci embody the archetype of the morally arrogant scientist over-reacher. The earliest recorded version of this archetype is the Biblical Nimrod, the great hunter and architect of the tower of Babel in the Book of Genesis. Fauci may have committed a Faustian-Nimrodian over-reach legally, as well as morally, in that he appears to have financed the Chinese gain of function research in stealth to evade President Obama's clear interdiction. One wonders, is there no limit to the arrogant presumption behind Fauci's scientific over-reaching?

Covid 19 was far from the first time Fauci, FDA, and the DTLM obstructed access to potentially life-saving drugs in order to pursue instead organizationally ambitious research agendas. It happened throughout the AIDS epidemic, a travesty I have documented in my book *How AIDS Activists Challenged America and Saved FDA from itself.* As I mentioned previously, the book shows that FDA and Fauci turned a blind eye to the illegal underground manufacture and sale of a drug, ddC, for which FDA did not want to grant accelerated approval. They shirked their duty to enforce laws that protect patients from illegal, defective, and potentially dangerous products in order to reduce community pressure on themselves to approve a legitimate and useful drug in a timely manner. AIDS of course is far from the only disease group with serious complaints against the deadly consequences of FDA delays. Examples are rife with cancer and many other fatal diseases, and especially with rare diseases. The imperial FDA strives to regulate everything that enters the human body. With the odd exceptions for sexual fluids, FDA seizes every chance it gets to extend its regulatory reign.

Tales of the frustrations, sufferings, and deaths of patients because of FDA delays in approving new treatments motivated Congress to pass the Right to Try Act of 2017. The Act was championed by Senator Ron Johnson and strongly endorsed by President Trump. It created a much needed safety valve, but without eliminating the root difficulties with dilatory FDA drug review and approval procedures. It left intact a hidebound bureaucracy administering a profoundly flawed system in desperate need of more fundamental reforms. We can only hope that the Republican nominee for President in 2024 will fully grasp the serious violations of individual rights inherent in current FDA drug approval delays as well as the gravity of the threats to public health an unreformed FDA poses in times of pandemic. The next nominee, along with the GOP itself, must make a firm commitment to far ranging transformation of this sclerotic agency. Otherwise, as the saying goes, history will repeat itself.

****

It is sheer speculation, one might argue, that had Dr. Fauci and FDA been over-ruled, or better yet if Trump had been able to reform FDA and put Fauci out to pasture years before Covid, and if our government had sensibly encouraged and facilitated use of the preventatives like vitamin D and zinc as well as alternative treatments like zinc combined with doxycycline and ivermectin or hydroxychloroquine, treatments where the evidence for their efficacy appears to be more substantial than the evidence for the preventative value of common forms of public masking, then those measures might have saved countless lives. That is what they appear to be doing where they are being used today in areas within Mexico, Peru, and India. We might also have kept the schools and much more of the economy open, thereby limiting the financial fallout from the epidemic.

We will never know because we didn't try it. No prominent official in government dared even suggest considering these measures—they were all too intimidated by the hallowed Dr. Fauci, the unassailable authority of the almighty FDA, not to mention the combined lobbying clout of the entire DTLM Complex. If that weren't enough, all knew that Google, You-Tube, Facebook, Twitter, et al stood ready to ban, sideline, or de-platform any who dared question the wisdom of the Great Fauci or the authoritativeness of FDA and CDC diktats. In retrospect, the failure of the media to probe about Fauci's and the FDA's opposition to the alternative treatments seems shocking moral cowardice, and a gross betrayal of professional ethics. How can the DTLM opposition to a treatment possibly be justified when the treatment is clearly safe, which cannot be said unequivocally of the Covid vaccines? Safety is relative of course, every drug, every food product has side effects. In saying the Covid alternative treatments are safe we mean as safe as commonly used drugs such as Tylenol or aspirin which have their side effects. Where were the media, the academics, the clergy, the doctors' organizations, the people's elected representatives? Not all were subject to DTLM-FDA intimidation, yet most remained silent.

Think about it. According to CDC at least 375,000 Americans died of Covid in 2020 before vaccines began to become widely available in January 2021. During that time hundreds of clinical doctors worldwide treating tens of thousands of patients witnessed to the efficacy of treatment cocktails with ivermectin or hydroxychloroquine used with zinc and doxycycline in early stage Covid. Yet the US government made no attempt to honestly investigate or test, let alone implement, these treatments. To the contrary, all FDA, NIAID, and DTLM efforts were bent on intimidating and slandering their proponents, urging the tech giants to ban them online, and otherwise impeding their use. How was this possibly justified when the cocktails were safe and no effective authorized treatments were available? If some doctors started prescribing vitamin C for Covid, would FDA have issued draconic safety warnings? They probably would not have done so, not because C is safer than ivermectin but because it lacks significant efficacy with Covid and therefore presents no competition to the FDA-DTLM's highly profitable vaccines.

Like good sheep, the country blindly followed the Great Fauci, the CDC, and our "authoritative" FDA who kept us in line by relentlessly fueling risk hysteria about the alternative treatments while disregarding the massive evidence for their safety and the mounting data supporting their efficacy. Instead they kept us busy mandating clothe masks they privately knew were in most cases close to useless and which they themselves donned only when the cameras turned their way. They distracted us with lockdowns they knew inflicted enormous collateral damage on the economy and the general public, damage from which their privileged lives were exempt. All the while they focused the vast resources of the Federal government on developing vaccines, something the DTLM would own and make hugely profitable. Although the vaccines are saving many lives, they have come too late for the hundreds of thousands who were discouraged or prevented from trying the alternatives that might have saved their lives.

****

'We know about Dr. Fauci and the FDA,' some might object, 'but where is the devil?' The devil is in the details, as the old saying goes. In this case it's the details of FDA restrictions, procedures, and propaganda that impede innovation by exaggerating risks and inhibiting accurate assessment of them within their context of risk filled human lives and in terms of risk/benefit tradeoffs. Panic is the primitive human response to the appearance of a serious threat to our physical persons or our survival. Once our flight impulse kicks in, we don't pause to calculate the likelihood that the threat will actually materialize.

Risk hysteria panics us into zero risk tolerance, regardless of cost. Zero risk or near zero risk always carries an exorbitant price tag in terms of costly tradeoffs. We could reduce our risk of dying in auto accidents to near zero by making cars so sturdy their occupants would survive nearly any crash, but such tank like cars would be prohibitively large, heavy, expensive and no fun to drive. Or we could impose a 30 mile per hour speed limit everywhere which would greatly reduce fatal accidents at the cost of massive increases in traffic gridlock and extra hours wasted on commuting. Rational calculation of risk, as opposed to risk hysteria, requires careful analysis of tradeoffs, like the collateral damage from the Covid 19 lockdowns, gratuitous school closures and school masking, damage that Fauci, CDC, FDA, and the DTLM complex either downplayed or judiciously ignored.

With drug approvals, the major risks of delay are born by patients who urgently need better treatments. The risks of accelerating treatment approval, the fallout from premature approvals, is born by FDA careerists and the clinical researchers who are blamed if anything serious goes wrong. That puts the patients' survival interest in direct conflict with the interests of FDA bureaucrats. Congress should have balanced the power to make decisions on access to new treatments more evenly and fairly between patients and regulators. Unwisely, it put that life and death power solely in the hands of the career bureaucrats. To do otherwise might have required thoughtful construction of independent oversight mechanisms, a task at which Congress has rarely excelled. So FDA and its' accomplices, like Dr. Fauci and the entire DTLM, were left free to prioritize the risks to themselves, which they routinely did, often at great cost to individual patients in desperate need of new treatments.

However, FDA, Fauci, and the DTLM give us an opposite narrative. They pretend their prime consideration is not their own interests but the interests of patients as group. Self-righteously reprimanding all criticism, they expect us to treat them as saints who would never dream of putting self-interest first. To distract from their calculated shifting of risk from themselves to individual patients desperate for new treatments, they generate risk hysteria about new treatments. They magnify the potential risks of treatments into hulking bogey men, and inevitably parade out those seventeen deformed thalidomide babies to march before us like terrifying specters in a horror movie. Yet like most bogey men, FDA fabricated risks, as in the cases of hydroxychloroquine and ivermectin, are wildly and dishonestly inflated to the point where they become ruses fashioned to manipulate and exploit the hapless, clueless, yet innocent public and dupe the sensation hungry media.

****

One wonders if bureaucrats like Dr. Fauci and his lifer cronies in FDA might have given Karl Marx or Fredrick Engels cause to reconsider trusting communist party bureaucrats to transform society and alter human nature for the better. Is it possible that in our time they might have seen the devils in the bureaucratic details of FDA procedures and plodding Fauci style research, or with their counterparts in China, and turned the focus of their activism from capitalists to unaccountable bureaucracies run by callous, mindlessly self-serving bureaucrats? They were certainly smart enough to grasp the problems bureaucracies pose. But Marx was German, Germans love order, and bureaucracy demands and instills order. However, Marx also strove consciously and unconsciously to represent and champion the lighter protesting Promethean aspect of the "bad boy" side of Jung's key hostile brothers archetype. The Marxist parties when they are able to seize power embody the grand contradiction in Marx himself between his German love of order and his Promethean drive to overthrow unjust order. Indeed, Marxism contains the seeds of its own destruction in the contradiction between its demand for order under party rule and its revolutionary impulse to overthrow order when it violates justice to chosen groups.

If Marx himself at least strived to manifest the lighter side of Prometheus, who, then, represents the darkest, totally corrupted Satanic aspect? My candidates would be the modern totalitarian bureaucracies, Marxist and otherwise. Dr. Mengele is a spectacular embodiment of the Satanic side. Yet Satan is not at his most effective and insidious when appearing as a grand, hugely inflated embodiment of evil like Dr. Mengele or his demented Fuhrer. It is Satan in the form of the snake, the affable, smiling, seductively benign yet ever cagey lying tempter, Satan the gelid bureaucrat, that is at his best in misleading and irreparably harming hapless humanity. The reader can guess the prominent contemporary examples I have in mind.

The Prometheus archetype that Marx saw as his personal inspiration boldly protests and confronts evil. But Satan and totalitarian minded bureaucrats, often clothed as harmless garden snakes, protect and enable evil by disguising it as something good and true; as St Paul warned:

> *for Satan himself is transformed into an angel of light.*
> *Therefore, it is no great thing if his ministers also be*
> *transformed as ministers of righteousness. 2 Corinthians 14-15.*

The corrupt bureaucrat always poses as the defender of the public's welfare. Yet it is all pretense, he seldom acts, never risks, let alone sacrifices himself or his bureaucracy for the common good of society let alone humanity. For him or her, the only goods that really count are the good of the bureaucracy and above all their own good as ambitious bureaucrats. CYA (cover your ass) is the golden rule for successful bureaucrats like Fauci and his fellow kingpins at NIH, CDC and FDA. This pattern is clear in the unfolding story of Fauci's and his colleagues' cover ups of their complicity/collusion/cooperation in the Chinese gain of function research that may yet prove to have been responsible for unleashing the Covid 19 virus on an unwary, excessively trusting humanity.

By its nature bureaucracy tends to instill an amoral totalitarian code, the Eichmann ethic, that slowly infects and corrupts the societies it rules. The paramount moral icons of West and East, Socrates, Jesus, and Buddha, teach an ethic that elevates our obligations to individuals, humanity and the truth over obedience to the state. Bureaucrats are trained to put first their obligations to their bureaucracy, which is usually an extension of the state. Bureaucracies, which pay and promote, their bureaucrats, insure that it is in these bureaucrats' interest to put the bureaucracy first. The Eichmann ethic, or the bureaucrat code, is atavistic, it is pre-Aeschylus, pre-Socratic, pre-Buddhist, pre-Christian and essentially Pharaonic. Its paradigm is the absolute obedience slaves "owe" their masters: bureaucracy is the Pharaonic, totalitarian adaptation of the tribe to a complex urban slave system. What is a slave but someone whose time and movements are owned and determined by another? As Orwell shows in *1984,* modern totalitarian bureaucracy surreptitiously re-institutes slavery by making all of us slaves to Big Brother, the modern image of the Pharaoh who personifies the original totalitarian bureaucracy. Every totalitarian regime ends up constructing slave camps, Hitler had

Auschwitz etc., Stalin the Gulag, and the CCP has its re-education camps
for the Uyghurs.

The Jesus of the Four Gospels courageously, if inconveniently for
the church bureaucrats appropriating his name, challenged the
bureaucratic tyrannies of the religious hypocrites of his day. John Milton
in his brief epic, *Paradise Regained,* underscores this feature of Jesus's
ministry by dramatizing his desert confrontation with a disguised Satan.
What does the tempter offer Jesus? Command of the greatest bureaucracy
of his day, the Roman Empire!

> *All of these which in a moment thou behold'st*
> *The kingdoms of the world to thee I give;*
> *For giv'n to me I give to whom I please,*
> *No trifle; yet with this reserve not else,*
> *On this condition, if thou wilt fall down,*
> *And worship me as thy superior lord,*
> *Easily done, and hold them all of me;*
> *For what can less so great a gift deserve?*
> *Paradise Regained, Book IV, 162-169.*

Milton's Jesus, who sojourning in the desert has deepened understanding
of himself, discerns and spurns this offer of bureaucratic power and pride:

> *Get thee behind me Satan, plain thou now appear'st*
> *That evil one, Satan, forever damn'd. 193-194*

Milton, himself one of history's greatest champions of liberty,
well understood the conflicts between conforming to the dictates of
worldly bureaucracies and the over-riding Christian duty to follow the
Golden Rule in respect to one's fellow man. Milton's Satan, the supreme
empire building bureaucrat of the Christian universe, offers Jesus the
greatest earthly prize bureaucracy can confer, command of the world's
government—in exchange for his soul. Unlike Dr. Faustus, Jesus is not
tempted to pay that price. Yet most contemporary bureaucrats readily, if
unthinkingly, pay Faustus's price when they blight and destroy other lives
with Adolf Eichmann's excuse, the bureaucrat's mantra, "I'm only
following orders."

What might Carl Jung have to say about Dr. Fauci, FDA, risk hysteria, and the massive socio-politico-medical-economic Covid crises in which we are mired? A Jungian approach attempts to transform the entire perspective of individuals so that they learn to probe the psychic sources of their own motives, recognize and curb ego inflation, and, where necessary, reject or even challenge bureaucratic authority in service of truth and humanity. Above all it can teach us to reject convenient/ expedient groupthink as a betrayal of our true self and of our moral responsibilities to other individuals. Instead, it turns to that self for guidance. Jung would seek a rejection of groupthink by the majority of humanity. Humanity itself must be transformed. Impossible some might argue. Yet both Carl Jung and Karl Marx, the two great opposing intellectual icons of our troubled era, ultimately advocated for a transformative change in humanity or at least human culture.

Humanity has adapted before, that is how we evolved from the apes. A world transforming cultural adaptation occurred when man moved from hunting and gathering to settle down on farms and build villages and then cities and civilizations. Another was the birth of philosophy and the civilizational religions in the era of those great teachers, Moses, Lao Tzu, Zoroaster, Buddha, Confucius, Socrates, Plato, and Jesus. It happened yet again with the rise of science and technology, and of technology's stealthily dangerous step child, the modern bureaucracy. So humanity, or at least human culture, can and does adapt. Our overwhelming question now is: will democratic Western societies wake up and adapt anew to overcome the ever growing abuses of bureaucracy, abuses that we've see writ large during the Covid pandemic with Dr. Fauci, FDA, and the DTLM complex?

Or will bureaucratic abuses powered by technology lead us down the broad expressway to a *1984* horror show where warring totalitarian behemoths clash by night? In short, do we continue to follow lemming like the bureaucratic devils leading us into the sea? Or, like Milton's Savior, will we identify evil, confront and reject it, and finally defeat it through deepened understanding of ourselves? Transformation or death, those are the alternatives for our age.

Chapter 4

Surviving the Woke Wake of Covid

You never let a serious crisis go to waste. And what I mean by that it's an opportunity to do things you could not do before.
*— **Rahm Emmanuel***

Politically, economically, and socially, Covid 19 opened Pandora's box unleashing myriad evils on a grievously ill-prepared world. As America emerges out of the most impactful pandemic since the bubonic plague periodically ravaged Europe, our social, political, and foreign challenges have become ominous, and our economic prospects are fraught with uncertainty. The problematic figure of Anthony Fauci, our ages chief incarnation of the archetypal Dr. Faustus, has become an emblem or icon (and to some degree an actual cause) pointing at the bureaucratic sources of our intellectual perplexities, moral mayhem, and societal upheaval.

The ugly self-serving mentality, prevalent in the DTLM Complex, that motivated FDA bureaucrats to ignore prophylaxis and block inexpensive mitigation treatments for Covid, and has long afflicted cancer treatment, may turn out to have cost hundreds of thousands of lives and inflicted untold economic and psychological damage. The DTLM will do its best to insure that we will never know for certain. Notwithstanding, America needs to recognize and grasp what happened, and who is at root responsible for the myriad mistakes with the Covid epidemic. Then we need to mete out public exposure and punishment where it is due. What we have seen so far is massive, systematic cover ups facilitated by big tech and their Woke political allies working in service of the DTLM. As a result, the misdeeds and the real and possible crimes of the DTLM have infected our political life through Covid. Transformational reforms are needed if America is to avoid descent into a steep curve of political, moral, and even technological and scientific decline.

Times of widespread chaos and massive corruption often follow civilization traumatizing events: US examples are the Reconstruction era during the Presidencies of Andrew Johnson and U. S. Grant after the Civil War, or the 1970s after the Vietnam war and the Watergate scandal, or to a lesser extent the Roaring 20s and Prohibition. We appear to be entering a similar time hit by 2020's triple whammy of the Covid pandemic, Woke riots across our cities, and a hotly disputed Presidential election.

While President Biden talks of uniting the country, he offers not reconciliation but only unremitting antagonism toward his political opponents which they often return with a vengeance. Instead of reaching out to them and to the moderates in between, Biden has fallen back into the clasp of the Woke extremists who appear to have hijacked the Democrat party. The extremists include Woke sociopaths, common in the Antifa and BLM movements, who assume absolute moral superiority, and that they are justified in using any and all means to retain and extend their power. True believers, these Wokesters want no dialogues or compromises; they seek instead to intimidate opposition into impotent silence where, isolated, it can be readily destroyed.

The sheer frivolity and vacuity, indeed the underlying sociopathy, of many of the Woke policies, if violent, mindless outbursts of sheer spite can be called policies, is breath taking. For example, in regard to enforcement of our border with Mexico they appear to be guided by no principle other than what I call their FYT rule----F**K YOU TRUMP. In this case, it means spitefully changing all immigration policies to be 180 degrees opposite to Trump policies regardless of consequences for American citizens.

All who cross the border illegally, after first paying their obligatory toll to the Mexican narcotics cartels, are treated as victims of iniquitous Trump policies and welcomed with open arms. Not always checked for Covid, all, regardless of Covid status, are handed bus or airline tickets to distant parts of the US where they may be given free housing, public assistance etc. Who knows what happens to them when the media won't do its job? Of those who are offered Covid vaccination up to one third reject it, yet they too are released with the others and free to spread Covid across the country which is exactly what they are doing. An estimated 18% of all these illegal entrants are infected with Covid, and some with new strains not yet present in the US population. They may well precipitate the next wave of the US epidemic.[32] While President Trump probably saved untold of thousands of American lives by stopping air travel to China, part of President Biden's legacy may be the thousands of Americans who will die because Biden opened our border with Mexico to tens of thousands of Covid infected people, many with dangerous new strains of the virus.

What do our chief guardians of public health, Dr. Fauci and the CDC, have to say about this massive, completely avoidable Covid danger? —nada, nothing, zero, zip, zilch! Their sheer irresponsibility is absolutely astounding. If Fauci had an ounce of integrity or courage in his little body, he would resign in protest, ditto for his CDC comrades. But wait a minute! Dr. Fauci and the CDC have an iron clad excuse, they were just following orders from the White House, Adolf Eichmann style. Besides, Dr. Fauci has a very busy schedule. Right now he's holding his third press conference of the day to lambast that annual Sturgis Motorcycle Rally in South Dakota. We can't expect a man with such important duties to find time to bother about a few tens of thousands of Covid super spreaders being shipped out to all fifty states, spreading their disease from sea to shining sea. Give the old doc a break!

Seriously, it makes you question the sanity of Fauci, those government officials like him, and those in the media who defend him. Are they really latent sociopaths analogous to people with walking pneumonia, in their case a walking psychosis that neither they nor others recognize and therefore become silent spreaders of their blight? How can a truly sane person not be troubled by the contradiction of turning a blind eye to loosing throughout the country Covid infected migrants, while focusing on a gathering of motorcyclists who decline to wear face masks, which are of all but useless and could be dangerous when riding a Harley? Has Fauci never heard of the principle of equal protection of the law, does he not realize that it means equal, or unbiased, enforcement of the law? Or has he violated equal enforcement for so long and so habitually it means nothing to him?

Along with Covid spreaders, criminals and terrorists are also welcome to cross our southern border. All that is required is to pay off the cartels who under Biden have become America's de facto immigration service. We even fly in at taxpayer expense the families of the illegal migrants without determining either their Covid status or if any of them are entitled to refugee status. We are bringing back those deported for entering illegally under Trump, as if everything illegal under Trump deserves to be extolled, legalized, and richly rewarded. If Trump deported them, they must be just the kind of immigrants we want! It's the wild, wild west wherever your umbrella policy is FYT spite.

Meanwhile, across the globe millions of responsible, law abiding potential citizens wait for years, often in vain and often in terrible circumstances, ready, willing, and able to obey our laws, and hoping and praying to enter the US legally. Cubans fleeing tyranny are shunned. Refugee camps across the planet are filled with displaced people with no lives and no futures, but we ignore their heart-rending cries and gut wrenching situations to give preference to whoever can pay the narcotics cartels to transport them over our southern border. It has become easier for a criminal or terrorist to enter the Joe Biden's US illegally than it is for many native born US citizens to return to their own country thru Covid wary TSA. How can you explain all this other than as a glaring instance of the sociopathic left's spiteful F**K YOU TRUMP uberpolicy?

Our border with Mexico is not the end but only the beginning of mind boggling irrationalities. The Biden Administration has turned Covid policies entirely over to Dr. Fauci, the DTLM Complex, and the teachers' unions, just as they forfeited control of the border and selection of new US immigrants to the Mexican narcotics cartels and their allied American sex trafficking gangs. If that weren't enough, they top it off by abandoning Afghanistan to the Taliban who are rushing to re-establish that country as a haven, sanctuary, and base for terrorists targeting the US, Israel, and the rest of the civilized world. The American people appear to be realizing that the Biden Afghanistan policies are tantamount to a self-inflicted Pearl Harbor. Because DTLM, the media, and big tech control what they learn about Covid, they are slow to recognize that the Biden-Fauci Covid policies are also a self-inflicted Pearl Harbor.

Perhaps to instill social regimentation and political conformity, the Biden Administration aggressively pushes masking far beyond whatever limited medical usefulness it may have. Education to persuade more people to get vaccinated is a good thing, but Dr. Fauci and the DTLM go further in favor of government compulsion, which the Biden Administration embraces and the left demands out of its sheer love of compulsion for compulsion's sake. The left's cancel culture warriors stand ready and eager to smear and then cancel any and all who voice opposition to mandatory masking and compulsory vaccination.

Besides F**K You Trump, the Biden Administration's ruling priority appears to be the Green New Deal imposed by Woke neo-Marxists who have hijacked the once sensible Democratic Party which they have altered beyond recognition in respect to the party of FDR, HST, JFK and even Bill Clinton. This is not the place to delve deeply into the irrationalities of climate fanaticism propelled through the Woke hijackers' determination to use the climate threat, as they use the threat of Covid, to extend government control over the personal lives of American citizens. Nor is it the place to review the jejune inanities of AOC, the Woke left's philosopher-in-chief and youthful, distaff parody of Anthony Fauci. Just as Fauci stands for indisputable "scientific" dogma, AOC stands for indisputable ideological dogma. Although in a free society science should never be dogmatic and neither science nor ideology should ever be indisputable. But don't try to tell that to the cancel culture warriors.

However, let me note parenthetically that environmental degeneration and destruction is a very real threat to the survival of civilization and humanity itself. Nonetheless, climate change caused by greenhouse gasses is only one factor and possibly not the most important. Pollution of all kinds, species extinction, and human overpopulation may well be or become more consequential components. Despite the lofty pronouncements of those heroes, seers, and saints of the left, lion hearted AOC, sagacious Greta Thunberg, deep thinker Don Lemon, the noble minded Keith Olberman, and the already Beatified Rachel Madcow, factors that mankind cannot control remain the most important determinants of climate change. These factors are led by variations in solar energy which in the recent geological past has caused huge glaciers to advance and retreat over vast areas including half of North America and the entirety of Thunberg's Sweden. The demagoguery of climate fanaticism could not be more imbalanced, inconsistent, dishonest, and blatantly self-serving were it a pooled effort of Dr. Fauci, the CDC, the CCP, the FDA, George Soros, and the Taliban.

Then there is Critical Race Theory, or CRT, lethal whiteness and the full menu of reverse Jim Crowe discrimination and demagoguery that has been unleashed into the intellectual chaos and moral vacuum that accompanies the Biden Presidency. Spreading with the infective speed of the Covid virus as a kind of psychic analogue to that virus, CRT aims to become an unchallengeable doctrine governing wide areas of American life. Would-be totalitarians always ride to power on the strength of their unchallengeable dogmas, witness Hitler's anti-Semitism.

Taking its cue from religious fanaticism, CRT and Black Lives Matter instant mythology has made George Floyd a saintly martyr and his conservative counterpart Ashli Babbitt a wicked plotter of treason who helped spearhead the most perilous armed insurrection since the Whiskey Rebellion. To borrow historian Victor Davis Hansen's succinct summary of our national dilemma:

> A pandemic caused by the leak of a Chinese-engineered virus and its cover-up is cause enough for nationwide madness. But the spread of COVID-19 was followed by a. nationalized and often politicized "flatten-the-curve" quarantine that soon ensured a stir-crazy nation. . ..

> Next ensued the death of George Floyd and a subsequent 120 days of rioting, looting, and arson. The immediate costs were $2 billion in damage, over 25 deaths, 14,000 arrests, and a Lord of the Flies anarchy with no-go zones in our major cities. A McCarthyite frenzy followed, as remote-controlled America hunted down the supposed "racists" among us—while career agendas, personal grudges, and ideological hatred fueled the cancel culture.[33]

The victim groups change, but their champions remain the same: Woke hooligans and opportunists exploiting their "by any means necessary" Marxist politicized pseudo-ethics. We saw this baleful phenomenon and toxic trend writ large in the contrasting cases of George Floyd and Ashli Babbitt. The collective insanities and inanities that swept the nation after Floyd's shocking May 25 2020 death, along with the events surrounding Babbitt's still murky January 6, 2021 death, are symptomatic and symbolic of profound dysfunctions in American society that Covid 19 forced to the surface.

George Floyd was a drug addict who served multiple sentences for armed robbery and narcotics possession. In one of his escapades Floyd threatened the life of a pregnant woman by holding a gun to her belly. Floyd appears to have been murdered by an out of line police officer, although a drug overdose on a constitution weakened by years of drug abuse was an additional factor. Though the circumstances of Floyd's death were fraught with uncertainties, the horrifying video of that event sparked an instantaneous rush to judgment by the MSM, BLM, Antifa, the academic elites, and opportunistic politicians in both parties.

Ashli Babbitt, in contrast, was an otherwise innocent young woman who never harmed or threatened anyone, and who went to Washington DC to protest the ruin of her struggling business by the State of California's draconic masking mandates and Covid lockdowns. Her death, according to unconfirmed rumors, came at the hands of an out of line security officer employed by Senate Majority Leader Chuck Schumer. In contrast to Floyd's assailant, the officer has never been charged, and his identity had long been withheld, though it was possibly leaked in July 2021. Posts sympathetic to Floyd flooded the internet; posts sympathetic to Babbitt were removed from social media and the big tech search engines. Meanwhile, the FBI is launching investigations of anyone who might be thinking about defending Babbitt and her right to protest. Many of Babbitt's fellow demonstrators are still held in solitary confinement on misdemeanor charges. Whatever happened to the constitutional ban on cruel and unusual punishment?[34]

The contrasts are heavily political. Babbitt was white, Floyd was black; Babbitt supported Trump; Floyd is supported by Black Lives Matter, Antifa, student demonstrators, academics, and the Woke MSM. Both were victims of misjudgment and serious police misconduct, as such both of them deserve sympathy. But only Ashli Babbitt died demonstrating for a cause she believed in; she alone has a claim to being celebrated as a hero. Although at this juncture none dare call her heroic, lest the FBI come knocking. One can hope that history will vindicate her. Floyd and Babbitt's contrasting situations, however, raise an urgent question: What ethical standard dominates contemporary political life in America? Is it still the Judeo-Christian ethic founded on love and respect for one's fellow man; or have the teachings of Jesus, the prophets, Rabbi Hillel and the traditional Christian churches been supplanted by ruthless Marxist opportunism following and enforcing the manipulated passions of a woke mob? America needs to wake up and ask itself which standard it wants to shape our national character and future.

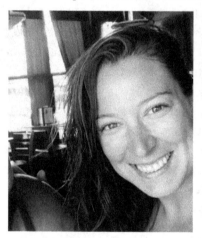 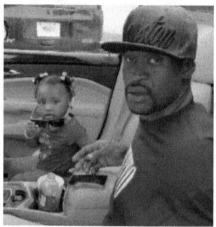

In the wake of George Floyd's shocking death and the disturbing events of January 6, 2021, advocates of critical race theory or CRT, saw an opportunity to seize the center of America's political stage. My many years as an advocate for gay and AIDS rights and my "standing" as an actual victim of anti-gay discrimination by the University of Wisconsin at Madison have given me a perspective on CRT that seems absent from the commentary and criticism I see in journalism today. The opponents of CRT make the mistake of dignifying it as if it were a rational system of argument that could be defeated by thoughtfully marshalling facts and reasons. My experience with another form of bigotry, homophobia, tells me otherwise.

You can no more defeat CRT activists by sound argument than you can thwart enraged bears, bulls, rattlesnakes or Nazis by trying to reason with them. Like Nazism, the KKK, and common gay baiting, CRT is not an argument but a mode of bullying and intimidation posing as an argument. It is actually unfair to traditional American Marxists to compare them to BLM and its Antifa allies. In that ideology's 1930's heyday, many, if not most, Marxists were actual believers who were sincerely deluded. Many left the movement disillusioned as more and more of Stalin's crimes were exposed. They were a different breed from the anti-Semites, Nazis, and KKK racists of the time who were pure opportunists with no stable beliefs. Ruthless determination to prevail was the racists prime motivation—their goal was Triumph of the Will, as in the Leni Riefenstahl movie title. They more resembled mobsters and gang thugs than religious or even ideological fanatics.

To understand today's self-styled Marxists, a good resource is Jean Paul Sartre's analysis of the anti-Semites of his time. Eclipsed by Marxists, Sartre and existentialism may seem passé today, but Sartre remains one of the most sociologically and psychologically insightful of all post World War II thinkers. Decades ago, I applied Sartre's brilliant work on the psychology of a racist bigot, *Anti-Semite and Jew,* to my analysis of Shakespeare's Iago. My dissertation advisor was a closeted homophobe who used my theory on Iago as one of his rationales for sabotaging my career in the teaching profession. I learned early by hard experience what motivates bigots, how they think, and feel. I paid a terrible price for my direct experience of bigotry, unlike the lazy, self-indulgent academic opportunists who have jumped on the reverse Jim Crowe CRT bandwagon to accelerate their career advancements.

Sartre's anti-Semite exhibits the passionate yet frivolous evil, the freely chosen malice unmotivated by real injury, that is commonplace in racism, homophobia, and religious and ideological fanaticism of all stripes. Sartre's percipient tract is all but forgotten today, yet its insights illumine the demagoguery behind our current racial dilemmas. Despite the frequency of discussion of racism and accusations of racism, we are afraid to examine the phenomenon critically lest we by chance step into some hidden pit of Politically Correct quicksand. We are eager to condemn generic racism broadly but reluctant to examine any particular form of racism. In our PC culture it is so much easier and safer to deplore racism and leave it at that. Sartre, writing before our dark age of PC, ventured beyond PC to dissect racist prejudice with the tools of an existential philosopher and psychologist. His trenchant analysis of the anti-Semite's core motivations, cited here in his own words, applies to bigots of all stripes. As an exercise, read Sartre's passage and simply substitute for anti-Semite whatever term you use for today's CRT, BLM, and Antifa reverse Jim Crowe "anti racists:"

> *The anti-Semite has chosen to live on the plane of passion. It is not unusual for people to elect to live a life of passion rather than one of reason. But ordinarily they love the objects of passion: women, glory, power, money. Since the anti-Semite has chosen hate, we are forced to conclude that it is the state of passion that he loves. . .. But there are people who are attracted by the durability of a stone. They wish to be massive and impenetrable; they wish not to change. Where indeed would change take them? We have here a basic fear of oneself and of truth. . . The anti-Semite has chosen hate because hate is a faith; at the outset he has chosen to devaluate words and reasons. How entirely at ease he feels as a result. . .. Never believe that anti-Semites are completely unaware of the absurdity of their replies. They know their remarks are frivolous, open to challenge. But they are amusing themselves, for it is their adversary who is obliged to use words responsibly, since he believes in words. . .. No one knows to what lengths the aberrations of his passion will carry him, but he knows, for this passion is not provoked by something external. . .. He has chosen to find his being entirely outside himself, never to look within, to be nothing save the fear he inspires in others.*[35]

Like Sartre's anti-Semites, the BLM, Antifa, CRT and Woke reverse Jim Crowe "anti-racists" have chosen, "to live on the plane of passion." To gain power and advance career opportunities, they have, like "good Germans" in the Hitler era, abandoned reason for passion, principle for expediency.

So how best to deal with them? The wrong way is to treat them as intellectually honest people who have simply reached incorrect conclusions. Give them the relevant facts and sound arguments and they will not for a moment consider correcting their errors and embracing the truth. No, they do not want facts or the truth, they want to win period. They have nothing but contempt for your facts, reasons, and truth, because they only display your ignorance of your vulnerable situation. Remember Marx said the goal of Marxism is to change the world, not to understand it. To win, to prevail, they are ready to use any means necessary. The change they seek is power for themselves, they will destroy anything to get it, including you. Trying to reason with them is like trying to reason with the Nazis trashing a Jewish store, with the hooded clansmen setting fire to an African-American church, or the knife wielding homophobes calling you faggot. How can you reason with that? You can't.

They are labelers, name callers, whose argument of choice is the *ad hominem* and whose aim is to humiliate and then bully you into submission. Their greatest strength is your inability to fully grasp what they are. They laugh the bully's cackle when you try to reason with them as if they were honest, reasonable people. All you can do is call their bluff: make it clear that you know their aim is to intimidate, but you refuse to be bullied. Gay leader and icon Harvey Milk once told me in a situation where he and I were literally being bullied physically by a pair of belligerent homophobes, "Never back down to bullies. Just remember when you stand up for yourself, you stand up for everyone like you." That is the proper moral position when facing bullies, whether they call themselves anti-Semites, white supremacists, or CRT anti-racists.

You defeat the CRT bullies not by argument but only by standing up to them. You must call them out for the shameless opportunists and amoral thugs they at bottom are. They are not essentially different from the KKK, the fag baiters, or the Nazis, all of them rely on lies and intimidation to get their way. The KKK's ultimate weapon was physical violence, the CRT bullies' ultimate weapons are verbal violence, labeling you a racist and using that label to intimidate you with the threat of destroying your reputation and thereby canceling you.

You must confront them by demanding respect and refusing to be bullied. Where intimidation boots out respect no discussion is possible. If you are a white or an Asian you should demand respect for the white or Asian human being you are and for the great European Christian, or Jewish, Islamic, Hindu, Chinese Confucian, or Japanese Buddhist, cultures you are proud to call your own. You must make it clear to them that you know their disrespect is the prelude to bullying and you are not about to tolerate being bullied. Remind them that their bullying is the essential tactic of racism, anti-Semitism, religious intolerance, homophobia and every other form of bigotry.

****

An ugly but ordinarily hidden truth about the political oppression of blacks in America is that with exceptions, like Martin Luther King, Thomas Sowell, Bayard Rustin, Harriet Tubman, Fredrick Douglass, and of course Barack Obama, blacks often allow themselves to become pawns rather than players in the power games of the whites' political factions. The terrible conditions of too many African-American neighborhoods, the crime, poverty, pollution, bad education in violent schools, and the deficient healthcare have continued since the 1950s despite African Americans' place as the pawns of choice in US partisan contention. CRT is a slightly novel tactic in the old game of leftwing partisan bullying, a tactic that cynically employs racist intimidation and crude ideology essentially similar to that of the Nazis or the KKK. CRT uses reverse Jim Crowe racism to empower Marxist demagogues who are often white and who pretend to serve the cause of oppressed blacks only to turn them into pawns in a political chess game that advances Marxism and the demagogues' own careers.

How to stop their malign game? Stable marriages, two parent families, and better jobs in the black communities would help enormously, but these solutions are more easily invoked than realized. What could be more readily achieved is school choice and empowerment of the parents who pay for the schools through vouchers. Parents must not only be allowed to choose their children's schools; they must be given a voice in regard to the curriculums their children are taught.

A second major step would be to stop the illegal immigration of poor, unskilled workers who compete directly with unskilled, impoverished black and Hispanic citizens lowering their wages and chances to rise while weakening the safety net upon which all of our poorest citizens depend. Either of these steps could be undertaken quickly; they would require only the will to do the right things for disadvantaged

Americans of every race, color, and creed. For the sake of the nation as well as for African American and Hispanic voters, Republicans must make these steps a center plank of their next campaigns. The chief opponents of school choice, the teachers' unions, have left themselves vulnerable by their destructive and unpopular school shutdowns. Republicans must push this advantage to the hilt, or lose it and lose our public schools systems forever. As for the Democrats, they must start putting the interests of their own voters and the country above placating Marxist Woke ideologues bent on winning by any means possible.

We search in vain for coherent, responsible immigration, environmental, educational, racial, energy, healthcare, or Covid policies where militant Wokism, the Squad, and F**K You Trump rule the field. All of these play out against a background of accusations of massive corruption involving Biden family deals with China, Ukraine, Mexico et al, and the antics of the all licensed Hunter Biden, the most problematic of Presidential offspring. Not to mention Biden's Afghanistan disasters and his desperate attempts to resurrect the nuclear agreements with an Iran that no longer welcomes them and remains pledged to the destruction of Israel and America. Besides these, there is more mundane madness like the canceling of the US Keystone Pipeline along with the Federal cut off of oil and gas exploration in the US. Following on the heels of this cut off, a major factor in rising US gasoline prices, Biden greenlighted the Russian Nordstream pipeline to Europe which enriched and empowered Vladimir Putin whom the same Joe Biden in his next breath denounces as a "killer." These acts move beyond the big spin to the much bolder "F**K YOU TRUMP" which becomes a mere corollary to the underlying principle of Woke sociopathic politics, "F**K AMERICA!" or to borrow from a Woke star of yesteryear, "God damn America!"

How to defeat them? You must stand up to the bullies. If you stand up, others will join you. But one brave, heroic person must always be the first to stand up.

The Woke hijackers of the Democrat party are financed by Soros and the corporate Swamp; take away their megabucks funders and BLM and Antifa will soon fade. Their funding will remain only so long as these groups are useful to help counter the threat of Trump reforms of the

Swamp. The corruption of the Woke left was foreshadowed during the AIDS epidemic as the FDA, Fauci, and the corporate DTLM recruited their cadres of shills to counter the threat of major FDA reforms posed by authentic patient activists and by then Speaker Newt Gingrich. Though the current Woke left has its new cancel culture, Fauci, FDA, and the DTLM have more practice and a longer history in canceling their critics. With the onset of Covid they upped their game of censorship in the name of "Science."

The DTLM's censorship path was blazed by the military industrial complex which thrived on vilification of opponents, fabricated threats, problematic wars, and unearned profits. A Big Tech Complex appears to be forming in the wings. Because of its information monopolies, and what it knows about each one of us, it threatens to become a more formidable danger to our freedoms of speech, press, communications, and even thought than the Military Industrial Complex ever was or the DTLM and the CRT "anti-racists" are currently. Notwithstanding, the potential of DTLM's monopoly on mind controlling drugs and gene altering technologies easily rivals Big Tech's threats to human freedom.

In post Covid America, the far right has its own absurdities to match the left; these pose dangers to our freedoms, especially because they can be used to rationalize further excesses by the Woke left. We must not forget Mike Pence and that sorry element in the Republican party which insists that teaching children that God wants homosexuals to be put to death, is a sacred right protected under the US Constitution's noble guarantees of religious freedom.[36] Or their insistence that the same religious freedom allows healthcare providers receiving tax funding to block medical information needed by women.

The greatest danger is not that so many of the accepted tenets and policies of the Woke left or the fanatic right are bad, though they can be very bad and destructive, but that we are becoming oblivious to the financial and moral corruption and intellectual vacuity in high places and have descended to routinely humoring political sociopaths and their demands. We have come to accept as normal politicians who subordinate every ethical principle to gaining, keeping, and expanding their personal power. Joe Biden or Mike Pence, it's six of one and half a dozen of the other. Since Ronald Reagan, America has seen a continuous lowering of the bar, morally and competence wise, for acceptable standards in its political life.

Anthony Fauci has become at once the emblem and court jester exemplifying the bankrupt integrity and moral vacuity that riddles politics in contemporary America. The Biden Administration is treating us to a *King Lear* reprise where Biden is the aging monarch with whom we constantly waver on whether to more pity or condemn his follies. Like Lear, Biden at bottom seems to want to do the right things. Yet, like Lear also, he is wildly volatile and easily manipulated into making terrible decisions that threaten to bring ruin to the realm. Biden has all of Lear's aged weaknesses and follies, some of his humanity, but none of his emotional grandeur or startling insight. In America's current surreal political drama of Shakespearean dimensions, Anthony Fauci alternates between the Machiavellian traitor Edmund (when playing opposite Trump) and the sycophant servant Oswald (playing opposite Biden). Alas, there are none in sight to play Lear's wise, compassionate fool. Where does this leave a bewildered, bedeviled American people and what will they do when they finally begin to grasp their dilemma in its full gravity?

Or what of Donald Trump, looming on the sidelines, like Fortinbras waiting to clear out the bleeding bodies left from Denmark's royal tragedy? Will Trump manage to return as did Charles De Gaulle, another extraordinarily difficult, problematic leader yet somehow capable of establishing a more viable order out of the pervasive chaos? Or will he return only to worsen the mess, a bringer of pointless, new chaos, like Juan Peron? Or will his star be eclipsed by someone like Florida Governor Ron DeSantis, lacking Trump's charisma but notable for bringing mind and mettle to the challenges of Covid and big tech? It all may depend on how well and how quickly the American people and Donald Trump himself grasp the royal mess we are in.

Will they see that the true culprits who created and perpetrated the disaster that is Covid are not Joe Biden, Kamala Harris, and their raucous crew of AOC, the Squad, BLM, and Antifa, who are mere trimmers and carpetbaggers. Will they recognize that the roots of their problems lie deeper with our criminally dysfunctional overlord bureaucracies, especially, in the case of Covid, the FDA and its allied bureaucratic manipulators of the DTLM complex led by the incarnation of Jung's ever inflated windbag, our Faucian age's archetypal Dr. Faustus? Will they realize that these in turn are but one large facet of America's uber problem with its overlord bureaucracies accountable to none but themselves, FBI, DOJ, CIA, DEA, IRS, et al? Will they understand that our revered Constitution provides no adequate mechanisms for oversight on our dangerous new overlords? Will enough people realize that we must find ways to make these bureaucracies accountable to the people, or else the people's freedoms will perish in the quicksand of totalitarianism?

Our overall challenge is to learn from our Covid mistakes, and we clearly have a lot of mistakes to learn from. We must do far better for the next pandemic which one day will come, perhaps right on the heels of Covid. While we don't know if there will be a major war or giant earthquakes, tsunamis, or game changing climate shifts in the lifetimes of our young millennials, it is all but certain there will be a next pandemic. Our crowded planet, our ever more intricately interconnected human community, our lack of effective, responsible government in too many regions combined with ever increasing biological experimentation done, without adequate oversight, for profit, or for bioweapons, or simply out of curiosity or by sheer accident, together these all but guarantee the creation and spread of new pathogens. Particularly dangerous would be an epidemic that starts as an act of bio-warfare, which Covid may actually be for all we yet know. Dr. Fauci may indeed know, but getting the honest truth from him recalls the old sayings about blood and stones.

At this relatively early point, we can still hope that any fatal leaks from the Wuhan lab were accidental leaks from a carelessly executed gain of function experiment that should never have taken place. That lab should not have been subsidized and participated in on the sly by US funded scientists, considering that President Obama had wisely forbidden such gain of function research. Somehow his interdict did not register with our era's over-reaching Dr. Faustus, who, by working around Obama's constitutionally binding orders, may well have become the epidemic's unknowing father. Evading constitutional authority has become the way of the world of the Swamp, especially proficient are the denizens of the

DTLM complex who hide their misconduct under the shield of "Science." When it comes to collusion, conniving, treachery, double-dealing, and duplicity, Big Tech could still learn a lot from the DTLM.

****

The virus as political weapon. In America today everything gets politicized, even a virus. The trend is not new in kind, it's a continuation from HIV-AIDS. What's new is its partisan intransigency. The war between the political parties on how to deal with the Covid virus, often exceeded in ferocity and commitment the war against the virus itself. For too many Democrats the great challenge became not how to defeat the virus, but how to exploit the pandemic in order to defeat Donald Trump.

America has long benefited from a two party system. We learned early in our history that a viable democracy requires multiple parties expressing diverse viewpoints and offering alternative solutions. One party cannot effectively represent everyone in a diverse, free society. Factions always seize control of the dominant party which inevitably becomes corrupted by its controlling faction. To retain control, they turn autocratic or even totalitarian. In a democracy, each party will make some grave mistakes; and so they will need to take turns at the rudder to keep the nation off the rocks. The successful resolutions to national problems often are those that best utilize ideas, draw on interests, and incorporate feedback from across the political spectrum. And that is why we need a free, broad, and vital political spectrum.

In the case of Covid the most serious mistakes, the most destructive policies, were disproportionately the work of Democrats— their arbitrary, heavy handed lockdowns that bankrupted small businesses, further enriched the superrich, and subjected many people to harmful social and psychological isolation, the paralytic and discriminatory school closures, the Democrat governors failures to protect nursing facility residents, the witless idolization of Anthony Fauci and his kneejerk kowtowing to FDA's sabotaging of re-purposed treatments, their resistance to scrutinizing the Chinese role in the genesis of the pandemic, their eagerness to enact draconic masking, and their readiness to excuse the FDA's and the CDC's delays in developing tests, guidelines, advisories, etc.---for all of these grave mistakes the Democrats have the lion's share of the blame. The onus of blame for Republicans falls chiefly on their failures to effectively counter and offer alternatives to the Democrats, and their decades of ignoring endemic FDA and DTLM abuses. Cognizant Republicans have long known that FDA is a dangerously dysfunctional bureaucracy, yet they have shirked the need for major reforms.

We had a situation analogous to the democrat's disastrous Covid policies with the parties reversed in the Iraq war a generation before. While some Democrats supported President Bush's wasteful, inappropriately motivated intervention in Iraq, the Republicans initiated it and bore most of the blame. Recognizing this, in 2008 the American people rejected John McCain, an Iraq war hawk, for Barack Obama who had vigorously opposed that war. Will the American people likewise grasp how the Democrats made the Covid crisis much worse by exploiting it politically and pin the tail on the donkey at the ballot box? They did not do so in 2020, in large part because of fanatical anti-Trump bias by the MSM and partisan censorship from the tech giants, such as their shocking election eve suppression of the Hunter Biden laptop scandal.

If the voters give the Democrat's possible crimes and clear mistakes a pass in 2022 and 2024, America's prospects will darken for dealing with the next pandemic more rationally, more ethically, and more effectively. The neo-Marxist Woke hijackers of the Democrat party would like to see America become a one party state, like New York and California appear to have become, or worse more like Venezuela or China. The Republicans must not let this happen. It remains unclear whether they and the American people are finally beginning to sober up from their Woke delirium to recognize the deadly threat that, once in power, Marxists will allow only one party, their own.

The Republicans failure to act on the recurrent and long-standing problems with the Swamp, FDA, Fauci, and the DTLM Complex may ultimately prove as destructive as the Democrats playing pandemic politics and exploiting racial divisions. Today neither party grasps that lack of oversight on the DTLM Complex forms a grave threat to America's security against pandemics. Neither realize that the DTLM, like the Military Industrial Complex before it, has no loyalty to anything beyond its own interests, or that its self-serving inflation of healthcare procedures and costs threatens to bankrupt the country, all the while denying its poorer citizenry quality healthcare. No major figure in either party, not even Donald Trump, is yet calling for investigation of the trouble fraught roles of the DTLM Complex, FDA, or CDC, or even the teachers unions. As of this writing Rand Paul has called for a DOJ investigation of Fauci. But no political leader has yet traced the problems with our pandemic preparedness back to their roots in the FDA bureaucracy and the excessive power that the 1962 Kefauver-Harris FDA amendment gave to FDA.

If the Republicans are to rescue America, as Lincoln and Teddy Roosevelt once did, they must have the grit to undertake major reforms of the country's educational, regulatory, and healthcare systems. A few understand this need, but a critical mass has yet to form. If the Democrats are to rescue America, as FDR and Harry Truman once did, they must recognize and repudiate Marxist thinking and methods, and re-instate allegiance to the Judeo-Christian ethic. They must also jettison their corrupting connivance with the FDA and other dysfunctional bureaucracies as well as with militant teachers' unions that ignore the needs and rights of students. The current situation in both parties offers scant hope that they will undertake the reforms necessary to insuring that in the next pandemic they will not repeat and amplify their mistakes with Covid 19.

Chapter 5

Vaccine Derangement Syndrome

In individuals, insanity is rare; but in groups
parties, nations and epochs, it is the rule.
— ***Friedrich Nietzsche***

Why have vaccines been viewed from the start as the preferred or even the sole solution to the Covid pandemic? Why not an array of defensive and offensive measures including treatments? When you go to war, you use your army, navy, planes, missiles etc., not just one of them. Follow the money. For the all-powerful DTLM Complex the big profits are in vaccines. There were no solid scientific reasons for relying exclusively on vaccines with Covid 19, certainly there was no reason not to run tests with existing meds: the decision to focus on vaccines was more based on DTLM economics and politics than on objective science. We could have focused on prophylaxis and treatments for Covid along with vaccines. But we didn't because the over-riding DTLM priorities are first and foremost maximizing profits (the companies) and second exploring research opportunities (Fauci's shop). If we save lives that's nice, but profits are what truly matters, and with Covid the big profits are in vaccines.

Similarly, during the AIDS pandemic in America voices were raised against developing treatments, and calling instead for the mono solution of vaccines. Some argued that treatments would be wasted on homosexuals who whose amorality made them responsible for their disease, but vaccines were needed to prevent the plague from spreading into the "innocent" general population. Others argued that the treatments would never work, they'd be too expensive and too hard to take regularly, and they couldn't stop the spread of HIV-AIDS in the minority populations. Still others insisted that the disease was not caused by HIV, Professor Peter Duesberg's criminal theory that killed patients who, because they believed it, refused HIV treatment. All were proved wrong. If these voices had prevailed with HIV-AIDS, and we had concentrated on vaccines and ignored the prospective benefits of treatment, AIDS would still be terrorizing American society. Why is it that here is probably the first place you've seen this critical point made?

We've spent vast sums on HIV vaccine research, and are still struggling to find a viable HIV vaccine, as we should. However, at the same time, due to unrelenting pressure from AIDS activists, we also developed drug cocktails that made HIV a manageable disease allowing its victims to live normal lives. Today there are 1.2 million people in America living with AIDS; their life expectancy is almost the same as that of the uninfected.

At the Covid pandemic's beginning, the DTLM and Dr. Fauci reached a silent consensus that this time *the* solution must be vaccines and only vaccines. With a heavy lift from Operation Warp Speed propelled by a very big boost from President Trump himself, three American companies developed effective new Covid 19 vaccines in less than one year. That condensed timeframe was unprecedented. Based on past vaccine development, Fauci, the FDA, and the rest of the DTLM initially projected that a vaccine would take three to five years. That is, if we had better luck with Covid than we have had for HIV-AIDS and hepatitis C. But viruses vary, for example we quickly developed new influenza vaccines every season, though they are usually only 30-60% effective, still they reduce the severity of the flu and so save many lives. We got lucky with the Covid vaccines and also, it seems, with the new mRNA vaccine technology. Next time we may not be so lucky.

Hi tech treatments like Regeneron were OK, they were patented and you could charge a bundle for them; but Fauci, FDA, and their DTLM country club buddies wanted vaccines first and foremost. Vaccines were the jackpot! What they did not want at all, no way Jose, was re-purposing old, cheap, unprofitable drugs to manage Covid by cutting hospitalization and death rates down to something close to what they'd be for a really bad seasonal flu. They claimed that if such drugs were approved and widely available, if you could cut the hospitalization and death rates by at least 70%, then the DTLM would lose support for developing their new types of vaccines for Covid. Their argument was flawed, and even dishonest, for several reasons.

There was no inevitable conflict between disseminating the inexpensive mitigation treatments, like an ivermectin based cocktail, and developing a vaccine: the need, the money, and the public support for both efforts was ample. As I pointed out previously, if some rules had to be changed to follow both strategies at once, we have a surefire mechanism for necessary rule changes, it's called Congress. We also have a second method, a Presidential waiver, and a precedent from when President George W. Bush waived FDA requirements in order authorize use of HIV rapid testing.[37] Because of the fear of Covid, the political will for the necessary changes would have been there in abundance—despite DC gridlock and Trump Derangement Syndrome.

Moreover, since not everyone will be able or willing to get vaccinated, treatment alternatives are essential to saving the unvaccinated. Given the degree of vaccine opposition across the entire globe, vaccinating the overwhelming majority of the human population is a pipe dream. Maybe North Korea can vaccinate their entire population. The nations of North America will not have that option, whatever Dr. Fauci, the FDA, and the DTLM bean counters may think or want.

Finally, the value of a treatment is relative to the severity of the disease, any drug that prevented death in 70% of advanced lung, pancreatic, or brain cancer patients would be considered a miracle and rushed through FDA, right? Think again. If the miracle drug were off patent, the FDA institutional culture would try to make those dying cancer patients wait for FDA to process a vaccine or a high tech new drug under patent, just as they blocked access to ivermectin forcing patients to wait for a vaccine.

Any way you look at it, the potential vaccine financial gains were irresistible to the DTLM. Where vast wealth was to be had, like the part time Woke Marxists they'd become, the DTLM bureaucrats and corporate magnates were ready to do "whatever it takes" to get every last dollar that universal vaccination promised.[38] The alternative treatments did not actually threaten vaccine development, but would pose a break on potential profits. If the FDA recognized alternative treatments, vaccines could still be recommended, but convincing the public that vaccines must be compulsory would become much more difficult. Most crucial, using the alternatives and limiting vaccines to individuals where the risk benefit ratio was favorable could mean a reduction of profits from truly humungous to merely gargantuan. Instead of hundreds of billions in excess profits, the vaccine makers might have to rest content with mere tens of billions. What a crushing blow to Pfizer and Moderna stockholders. Boo hoo!

Not ones to let a crisis go to waste, the DTLM Complex wanted to reach for the biggest possible jackpot. They duped themselves into a huge inflation by thinking, 'with no treatments available, if Fauci and FDA can raise a big enough scare, then we could justify vaccinating the entire human race, a market of truly unprecedented size and unique profitability.' Vaccinate everyone, and make hundreds of billions by doing so! Vaccinate everyone and add more sheen to the glitter of FDA's glorious gold standard! Vaccinate everyone and make Tony Fauci a world hero, more famous than either Taylor Swift or Le Bron James, on a par with the Queen, Donald Trump, and, hey, why not Jesus! —Just imagine our Tony sharing center stage at the big medical conferences with his three new best friends, Bill Gates, Jeff Bezos, and Mark Zuckerberg, (dear, indispensable Zuck!) standing respectfully several steps behind Tony of course! Or how about the Pope kissing Dr. Fauci's ring! —that's be one for the history books!

There was one little problem. A vaccine developed within a year could not be thoroughly tested for safety, such testing could take much longer. It would be one thing to vaccinate the world with a proven vaccine like that for tetanus, and quite another to vaccinate all of humanity with an experimental vaccine whose side effects, particularly the long term ones, were as yet unknown. That might have been justified as necessary with a much higher fatality rate, say 10% rather than Covid's mere 1%. A much higher fatality rate would have terrorized the entire planet to the point where it collapsed, rather than crippled, the world economy. Nonetheless, without processing through elected officials, without even apprising them of all the medical facts and options, the DTLM, through the FDA, CDC,

Dr. Fauci and their ever pliant media shills, began to manipulate the public to prepare for universal vaccination, exposing to unknown vaccine risks youths, children, and infants who are at much less risk of dying of Covid than they are from an ordinary seasonal flu.

President Trump, along with others who understand the world economy, knew we could not afford the three long years of the Covid panic and lockdowns that Fauci, the DTLM, and the Trump Derangement Syndrome Democrats seemed bent on generating. After three years the world economy would be a basket case, 1932 all over again! Then what? A 21st century Hitler wielding H-bombs? Tehran nuking Tel Aviv and getting nuked right back, with Karachi nuking New Delhi next? So three still experimental vaccines were approved, after only 9 months testing and development, to be used on the entire population of planet Earth. And it was approved with nary a whisper about any windfall profits tax---where were Bernie Sanders and Elizabeth Warren, napping in the rose gardens of that grand Bethesda mansion NIAID provides St. Tony?

Given that the Covid vaccines are all experimental, their safety hazards incompletely tested, given that for the overwhelming percentage of people under forty, with exceptions like diabetics and the morbidly obese, Covid is no more life threatening than the flu, given that for most people under forty the unknown risks of taking the vaccine may well outweigh the minimal known benefits, there is no conclusive medical justification for mandatory vaccination for everyone under forty. Vaccination for them should be an individual choice made in consultation with their physicians. However, for Dr./St. Fauci and the DTLM Complex two other justifications easily sidelined the most basic principle of medical care, "first do no harm" ---these were *profits and power*.

To maximize vaccine profits you need to maximize the market, that's simple economics. To insure that everyone would take the vaccines you need an entire population terrified of getting Covid, which is what FDA, CDC, Fauci, the DTLM and their counterparts across the globe set about doing from the onset. We were again treated to yet another exhibit of the tried and true FDA risk hysteria that's been hardwired into their institutional culture since thalidomide. Panic had another secret advantage dear to the fast beating hearts of St. Tony and the careerists at FDA, if not to the cold blooded DTLM bean counters—inducing risk hysteria and panic in the populace is their secret intoxicant. Forget opium, meth, heroin, and oxycodone, nothing sends them up like the sense of their own power. What an escape from their dull bureaucratic lives, that rush of supreme, arbitrary, institutional power over helpless, terrified mortals. It's the DTLM bureaucrats' answer to a crack cocaine rush!

And so from the onset, Covid panic became the order of the day. Wildly inflated projections of death rates from now discredited UK sources were touted by Fauci and the DTLM and amplified through the most massive megaphone ever constructed, the worldwide internet.[39]

President Trump prudently advised people not to panic, but given the pervasiveness of Trump Derangement Syndrome his warnings had just the opposite effect. If Trump says not to panic, cried his myriad detractors in the MSM and throughout the Woke left, that must mean we have very good reasons to panic. Or if we don't, let's do it anyway just for the hell of it! And panic they did. The one affliction that spreads faster and is even more infectious than Covid 19 itself is panic. Countries that were not in any serious danger of widespread epidemics, like Thailand, Australia, Vietnam, New Zealand, and Argentina, collapsed into panic like dominoes, all their schools in lockdown, their factories shuttered, their tourist industries crumbling as fast as dominoes fall. For the corporate DTLM bean counters, panic was just what the doctor called for. Panic insured a huge market juiced by powerful social and governmental pressures on everyone to get vaccinated.

Initially, pressure seemed necessary to bring into line a populace ridden with vaccine skeptics and vaccine paranoids. Skepticism was of course largely justified in respect to still experimental vaccines; indeed, skepticism is a wise and proper scientific minded attitude toward anything new, incompletely tested, and imperfectly understood. Moreover, the right to make your own choices, even if imprudent, or uninformed choices, is an essential feature of personal freedom. In financial matters of great consequences Americans ordinarily take risks that turn out badly, they buy the wrong house or car, or they pick investments that go south, it's called the free market. Indeed, Americans are constitutionally guaranteed the right to make a wide range of personal mistakes, however little the great

Dr. Fauci may esteem the exercise of freedom by the mendacious likes of a Sen. Rand Paul and his illiterate, hillbilly fly-over country constituents.

Fauci's undisguised contempt for Senator and doctor Rand Paul notwithstanding, Paul's vaccine reservations are sensible and science based given that the Covid vaccines are still experimental and lack long term safety data. While the vaccines long term dangers remain uncertain, they have already built an exceptional record of disturbing side effects, including some vaccine related deaths. I still suffer unpleasant side effects from the Moderna vaccine, yet for me at least, these painful side effects are balanced by knowing that the hastily developed, incompletely tested, vaccines have saved countless individuals from severe Covid infections and are enabling the rest of the population to resume normal lives.

So we had a situation where vaccine panic contended with DTLM induced virus panic. The DTLM knew vaccine panic could endanger profits, indeed vaccine common sense was an even greater danger to profits because it would insure that many of those under forty would decide that they lacked a compelling risk/benefit ratio for taking the still experimental vaccine. However, there were more profits and jobs at stake than just those within the DTLM. Because of the Covid panic and the crippling restrictions routinely imposed by blue state politicians seeking advantages in the 2020 election, the huge hospitality, airline, and tourist industries were on life support. Business travel and ordinary tourism needed to return to normal and workers needed to return to factories to bring the entire world economy back to life. The vaccines became the only way to insure that a virus panicked populace would feel free to travel again and return to work.

A failing world economy would mean millions dying of various forms of deprivation or despair, the most common being postponed or insufficient medical care, drug addictions, and suicide. Indeed, it may well be that the economic setbacks from the virus have so far killed more people than the virus itself According to various scholars, the Covid epidemic has driven hundreds of millions into poverty.[40] Thus, it might be argued that everyone has a moral responsibility to get vaccinated, even if their personal risk benefit/ratio is unfavorable, in order to help save the world economy and those suffering severe deprivations. That was a part of my thinking when I chose to be vaccinated. But I also thought and still think that individuals must be left free to make their own Covid vaccine decisions without external constraints. Free persons must at least own their own bodies, the term for persons who don't is "slave." If the government owns our bodies, then we are the government's slaves.

Most individuals are chiefly concerned with protecting themselves and their families. From that perspective, the vaccines are still experimental, and disturbing side effects are still showing up and may continue to do so over the next several years or even decades. We do not know how serious or widespread these side effects will ultimately be. One of the most frightening manifestations has been the cases of myocarditis in boys and young men in Israel. This is particularly tragic and truly outrageous because there is no clear medical justification for vaccinating healthy young men, or women for that matter—only a clear profit motive.

I received my first dose of the Moderna vaccine on January 20, 2021. I was 77 at the time and suffer from auto-immune disorders and a heart condition. But I do love to travel and wanted to do my bit to stop Covid, so taking the vaccine, risks and all, seemed an acceptable gamble. A week later I came down with a severe case of shingles, a painful, nasty affliction I had never experienced before. Seven months later the lesions have disappeared, but pains and constant itching along the afflicted lateral nerve persist. So far the side effects have not caused me to regret taking the vaccine, but I am concerned about what else this powerful, experimental vaccine may have done to my health. Nasty side effects like mine are not unusual. My dermatologist reported that among his patients a total of six cases of shingles appeared shortly after receiving the Moderna vaccine.

We don't know how many will ultimately suffer severe vaccine side effects or worse, although the casualties appear to be exponentially greater than with other well tested vaccines in common use. As yet, we know nothing of the long term effects of this new technology of mRNA vaccines. But what we have seen should make us cautious. Healthy younger people who reject the vaccines are not fools or sociopaths who deserve to be shut down online and canceled socially—contrary to what

Dr. Fauci, the FDA, the corporate DTLM, and the compliant tech giants might like us to believe.

Anti-vaccine censorship. All of these vaccine problems and fears taken together, are enough to give people prone to conspiracy theories sufficient fodder to pursue their passion for months on end. And so they do. Thanks, or perhaps no thanks, to the tech giants, the internet is not as full of Covid vaccine conspiracy theories as you might expect. The officious tech behemoths, sustaining members all of the Tony Fauci Fan Clubs of America and dogmatic, if blindly credulous, believers in FDA's "authoritative truths," severely restrict negative information on the vaccines to complement their knockdown of positive information about the treatment and prophylaxis alternatives/supplements to the vaccines. Tech censorship made informed individual decisions more difficult, and it inadvertently did as much to amplify as quell unreasonable fears and wild conspiracy theories.

The tech giants have gone so far as to ban the warnings against childhood Covid vaccination issued by the World Health Organization. Previously WHO was second only to the Holy of Holies, the FDA itself, in the techs' hierarchy of unfailing sources of "authoritative truth." The techs, it seems, can be as fickle as they are powerful, even though their caprices steer compulsively toward the left. It often seems like Lewis Carroll's erratic Red Queen reigns over Silicon Valley. The techs actions in the Covid pandemic and interference with the 2020 election inevitably bring to mind Lord Acton's famous maxim: "Power tends to corrupt and absolute power corrupts absolutely."

Medical misinformation can be a serious problem, but censorship creates far-reaching threats to individual rights, and personal freedoms. Censorship endangers innovation and the survival of democracy itself. Without censorship individuals are free to sort through information and misinformation to find the truth, or at least free to formulate and express their own opinions. Some will make mistakes, but that's their right, and hey, learning from mistakes has advanced human civilization along with the evolution of the life itself! However, the tech giants and their allies in the DTLM Complex, especially the FDA, often view novel information as a challenge to their authority and so they label it misinformation, even though they haven't a clue whether that label is correct or not. The individuals who run these tech corporations are free to make their own private assessments, but as common carriers their companies have no business denying that freedom to the general public. Censorship leaves the public with only the authorities' self-protective, self-serving views. Free thought, freedom of speech, information, and communication are all abrogated by censorship: without these freedoms, innovation, creativity, and progress die along with personal freedom. Without freedom democracy itself perishes; *freedom is democracy's raison d'etre.*

Chapter 6

The Science of Virology
meets the Art of War

The enemy is anybody who's going to get you killed,
no matter which side he is on.
— Joseph Heller, Catch-22

One lesson from Covid seems certain: in the future, we must treat pandemic challenges of Covid's magnitude as seriously as we would a war. Whether generated by deliberate acts of bio-warfare launched by a foreign adversary or terrorist group, or generated without human connivance by a natural organism, the stability of democratic societies is immediately threatened. The more complex and interdependent our society becomes, the more vulnerable it becomes to pandemics. A largely rural, agricultural society can much more easily withstand a population decimating pandemic than can a post-modern urbanized society where everything needed to sustain life, food, water, etc., must be provided by the economy, and where, because of high tech communications, panic can spread instantaneously.

A deliberate launch of a bio-weapon is more likely to happen now that Covid has shown the bad actors of the world how it could be done. Indeed, bio-warfare has become a more immediate and more probable threat than nuclear war. Retaliation with mutually assured destruction reduces the likelihood of nuclear war. Bio-warfare would be launched in stealth, destroying the enemy before he figures out who his attacker is. Given what we've seen totalitarians do, the holocaust, the gulag, Mao's cultural revolution, the killing fields, the Taliban, does any realist believe regimes like those of the Kims in North Korea or the Iranian Ayatollahs are incapable of taking a cue from Covid to pursue/achieve their goals of dominance? Once Covid 19 entered our populace we were at war with that virus. Call it a pandemic rather than a war if you want, but just like an ordinary war it created havoc in our economy and threatened the stability and even survival of our nation and civil society. Consequently, some war measures, such as Warp Speed, were appropriate and they will be appropriate for future pandemics. Nonetheless, protecting basic personal rights is always a challenge, and that is never more true than in wartime.

To avoid repeating our mistakes with Covid we must first recognize those mistakes, fully investigate them to assess responsibility, then condignly punish those responsible, and finally pass laws and develop policies to better protect America from future pandemics. The biggest challenge will probably be to recognize and acknowledge our mistakes. That will prove difficult because those responsible for the biggest mistakes, particularly Dr. Fauci, the FDA, and their cohorts in the DTLM Complex and the MSM, will remain in deep denial. They are certain to launch deliberate cover ups and spread misinformation to conceal their guilt from others and obscure it from themselves. We know they've already had plenty of practice in the arts and crafts of cover up and misinformation—it's the Way of the Swamp.

What salient mistakes with Covid can we identify at this early point? First, don't panic and don't use the adversary, e.g., a virus we incompletely understand, as an excuse for accelerating domestic political divisions and pursuing private agendas. When a country is attacked by a foreign adversary, it must unite to survive. We need to understand that a lethal virus is one of the worst possible foreign adversaries. Yet, like everything else in the era of Trump, the Covid 19 virus became highly politicized with Trump's opponents lambasting everything he did and said. Their hysterical reaction was off the charts with hydroxychloroquine, but equally unhinged was their stubborn opposition to ivermectin, and other prophylactic and inexpensive mitigation treatments. Those afflicted with Trump Derangement Syndrome in academia and the Pravda media, along with the Woke hijackers of the Democratic Party whose uberpolicy became "F**k You Trump," greeted Covid as yet another battlefield on which to combat Trump, public health considerations and the welfare of the nation and the world be damned.

The DTLM, bent on the golden Eldorado that the vaccines promised, opposed every attempt to explore preventatives like Vitamin D and zinc or to treat Covid infection at its onset with ivermectin or hydroxychloroquine. Trump's political opponents made things worse by seeing the DTLM's strategy not for what it was, a ruthless attempt to use the pandemic to profit and increase their power regardless of the cost in American lives, but as an opportunity to find allies and score political points against Donald Trump. America needs to recognize the motives of those within the mega money elite who are pushing Trump derangement syndrome. The biggest players are the mainstream news, the tech giants, and much more quietly the DTLM Complex. So far too few recognize the DTLMs amoral character or grasp its ominous power. Certainly, the DTLM is the most powerful and least understood player in the Covid crisis. Trump's attempts to revoke Obamacare and to restrain drug prices stirred the DTLM against him. With Covid the DTLM saw a golden opportunity to rid itself of the real and imagined threats posed by Donald J. Trump.

When a new pandemic first appears we must gather as much information as we can as fast as we can. To deliberately impede the flow of information about the disease and ways to treat or prevent it is morally equivalent to aiding the enemy in a war. From the start, FDA and CDC were at fault for letting bureaucratic sludge and rivalries slow the process of gathering, evaluating and disseminating vital information, such as the differences in vulnerability of various population segments, like the over sixty-five versus the under thirty.[41]

To impede or block information, from any source, domestic or foreign, that may be vital to our survival as a society facing a bio-threat should be a serious crime. Freedom of speech and communication are essential to finding solutions to every novel problem, nowhere is that more true than in a pandemic. Those who aid the viral enemy, especially for political or economic gain, are guilty of acts comparable to treason and may well deserve to be dealt with accordingly.

To insure that mistakes are more quickly revealed and acknowledged, we must stop honoring the "Eichmann out," the bureaucrat's threadbare excuse of "only following orders." Every bureaucrat that works for FDA, CDC, NIAID, NIH, as well as FBI, CIA, IRS, DEA, etc. has an over-riding legal and moral obligation to the United States of America, its Constitution, and its peoples; that obligation must always outclass obligations to their employer. This principle, however, is rarely, if ever, imparted to government employees who instead are encouraged to defer to their superiors "authoritative" understanding of the interests of our country and its peoples.

Whistleblowers must be encouraged and given effective protection from retaliation. Bureaucratic accountability is essential. We do not have it so far on Covid 19 or in most other areas of our public life. For example, as of this writing Dr. Fauci is still refusing to answer fully critical questions about the origins of the Covid virus posed by Republican Senators. We will have even less accountability next time if we fail to enforce accountability for the Covid pandemic. Though Washington commissions are often dismissed as empty political exercises, they can be a useful, even necessary, means to establishing and promulgating facts about past mistakes and misbehavior. They provide a platform for diverse points of view because it is more difficult to squelch dissent on a commission than it is within a typical bureaucratic hierarchy.

Like the Kennedy assassination, the Covid pandemic has profoundly disturbed our entire nation and raised urgent concerns about the possible involvement of foreign powers, specifically China. Conspiracy theories abound and proliferate in the absence of clear facts and solid explanations. As an essential step toward restoring confidence in government and healing America, we will need a new "Warren Commission" to investigate the origins of the Covid virus in China and any and all involvement of US citizens or agencies in its creation or dissemination. It is every bit as important for the American people to know what happened with Covid 19 as it was to know the truth about the Kennedy assassination. Unfortunately, records from that event are still withheld, which does not bode well for full disclosure on Covid.

We also need to investigate in depth the dogged resistance, indeed the sabotage, from FDA and its DTLM allies on using re-purposed treatments like ivermectin in early Covid disease stage. How did it happen? What was the genesis of the *Lancet* hydroxychloroquine hit piece? Why did they run their trials with patients in late disease stage when doctors who use this drug and ivermectin specify its use only for early stage? FDA has a sorry history of running "designed to fail" trials with vitamins and other supplements that it wants to trash. What were the actions, motives and complicities of key actors within the FDA and the DTLM Complex? What kind of culture prevails in the FDA that its staff seem to so readily assume the agency's interests outclass the interests and the constitutional rights of the American people? Did FDA employees engage in criminal or unethical behavior that needs to be investigated, prosecuted, or outlawed? These are questions that America will leave unanswered at its peril.

Particularly crucial are the clouds around Dr. Fauci and his associates in NIAID that obscure their cozy relationships with FDA and above all with the Chinese officials involved in Covid research linked to gain of function experimentation. Rand Paul has raised crucial questions and concerns about the Chinese bioweapons lab for which the American people are entitled to answers. How much in total did Fauci pay the Chinese to conduct the Wuhan gain of function experiments that Obama made illegal in America? Under what conditions was it funded, and what oversight, if any, was part of Fauci's deal? What do we have in documents such as contracts and proposals or emails? Who above Dr. Fauci knew about and approved the research, or was it basically a covert deal between Fauci and the Chinese? Fauci knew it was dangerous research; what precautions, if any, did he specify to protect the world from an accidental release of a dangerous bio-threat? He has made it appear as if he just handed them the research money carte blanche and knew almost nothing about what they might do with it. If it was not like that, what was Fauci looking for, what did he expect in return? As Desi Arnaz might have told Lucy, "you got some splainin to do."

Senator Paul appears to have opened a can of worms, or more likely a barrel of vipers. Many conservatives are quietly wondering, could Fauci be the 21st century version of a war criminal? —or is he merely an inflated over the hill bureaucrat who habitually lets ego cloud judgment and vanity misdirect his behavior? Either way Fauci should go. The most important thing he has to do at this point in his career is to show us what he knew and when, why he did what he did and who he did it with. Fauci's Covid press briefings should be left to the appropriate NIAID PR flaks where they should have been all along.[42]

The first really big mistakes with Covid 19 were not made in the Bethesda backwater of the DC Swamp, but where the virus originated in CCP ruled China. The Chinese government failed in its moral and legal obligations to give the world advance warning of a dangerous, novel virus they knew was on the loose. They aggravated the problem by their refusals to provide specific information on the virus once it had spread outside China. Careless Chinese researchers may have accidentally released the virus from their Wuhan bioweapons lab where the safety protocols were known to be sloppy.[43] What was not accidental was the Chinese decision to ban flights from Wuhan to the rest of China while allowing Covid infected Wuhaners to fly internationally to vacations across the world thereby infecting the world. A clear chain of evidence shows how these tourists initiated the epidemic that devastated Italy in early 2020 and soon spread to France and Spain and then across Europe and the world. Since then, recalcitrant Chinese officials have stubbornly refused to allow foreign researchers access to the Wuhan lab and its data.

Recent information confirms that the first Covid cases began to appear in Wuhan in September 2019, months before the start of the Italian epidemic in January 2020.[44] In all probability, China could have given the rest of humanity several months warning, but chose not to do so. However, the US and other nations failed to act expeditiously on January 2020 information flooding in from Italy, France, Spain, and other first stops for the virus. This provided very early data warning that certain population groups, especially the elderly, the obese, and diabetics, are far more vulnerable than the general population. We knew these vulnerabilities well before the virus began to get significant footholds here. Yet some states, such as New York, New Jersey, Michigan, and Pennsylvania, put Covid diagnosed patients back into nursing homes, at the ultimate cost of tens of thousands of avoidable deaths.

Republicans like to blame these state's governors who were all Democrats, but these governors share blame with the CDC and Dr. Fauci who failed to intervene aggressively on behalf of the nursing home residents. In any event, Biden's DOJ is declining to investigate the nursing home deaths, so neither these victims nor their loved ones are likely to ever get justice or even so much as the respect that would be shown through a conscientious effort to obtain an accounting. This again underlines America's need for a new "Warren Commission" to ascertain the truth about where the Covid 19 virus came from and who is responsible for the appalling mistakes that escalated the nursing home death toll, and other errors that worsened the overall epidemic and its collateral damage.

Throughout the epidemic many authorities have acted as if Covid 19 constitutes a serious threat to the entire population when from the beginning there was ample evidence that, for anyone under forty without underlying conditions, Covid is unlikely to be more deadly than an ordinary seasonal flu for which we take few special precautions. With Covid we needed to identify, protect, and if necessary isolate the most vulnerable. We consistently failed to do so because many in the DTLM and the political establishment sought to maintain the fiction that Covid was an imminent threat to everyone, thus rationalizing lockdowns and school closures that were often motivated more by politics than by immediate public health threats. With the DTLM the motivations were simple greed for wealth and power, their determination to maximize the market for their very profitable vaccines, and, especially in the case of FDA, their desire to maintain total control of turf. With the politicians, the motive was to win the next election at any cost, even the cost of thousands of human lives.

Far too little was done to protect the most obviously vulnerable groups led by the elderly over 75, but including African Americans, and native Americans. As one of the oldsters, I saw scant evidence of any serious efforts by the State of Nevada authorities to insure that the general public and private businesses were aware of or cared about our special vulnerabilities. All of the vulnerable groups might have benefited greatly from expanded efforts to educate them on simple available steps to improve their chances with Covid. Especially helpful would have been widespread information on the value of prophylaxis with vitamin D and zinc supplements, plus the option of prescribing early in the disease treatment cocktails based on repurposed ivermectin or hydroxychloroquine combined with zinc and doxycycline. But the Governor and state officials of Nevada did just the opposite, they went all out for the FDA spearheaded campaign to politicize and then discredit these treatments.

Another big mistake was the continuing bureaucratic snafus by FDA and CDC in getting out the Covid diagnostic tests. This needs further investigation, and those guilty of putting bureaucratic turf interests and unbending procedures above the need to protect human life should be identified and disciplined as appropriate. Given the current political climate, it is all but certain that nothing will happen, unless of course these snafus could be construed to fix the blame on white supremacists or, best of all, Donald J. Trump. Then the sleeping MSM would awaken screaming for blood.

As I have maintained repeatedly throughout, the worst mistakes may prove to be the DTLM-FDA led failure/refusal of Federal and local government agencies to identify and implement re-purposed treatments like ivermectin. Blame for this lies squarely with the culture of FDA and its incestuous relationship with the corporate DTLM. Fundamental change here would require drastic FDA reforms imposed by Congress and the President and backed by public understanding and voter demand. That's a tall order, but next time America's survival could indeed be at stake.

Behind too many of the Covid mistakes you will find "by the book" FDA careerists putting the interests of their hidebound agency and themselves first, keeping vital information from the public, floating misinformation about treatments they disfavor, manipulating the press and media, and usurping executive powers and crucial decisions that rightly belong only to elected officials. The FDA bureaucrats and Dr. Fauci in effect claimed a modern version of divine right, as if their vaunted authority came from their proclaimed secular god "Science." Although that attitude is risibly unscientific, no one in the mainstream media laughed, they took all too seriously the FDA overlords inflated claims to omniscient authority.

However, with Fauci and FDA, the ever shifting scientific data too often failed to support what they loudly asserted was "the Science." When the crucial data did come in, such as the median age of those who died of

Covid and the critical role of co-morbidities like diabetes and obesity, it was hardly so complex that it took a professional scientist to grasp its public health and ethical implications. Moreover, Fauci didn't always abide by what he believed to be the science, as we have seen with his emails expressing skepticism about the efficacy of the masks in common use.[45] In fact, his MO was to follow the politics over the science all the while equating himself with "Science." History shows that impressive credentials in science do not reliably indicate understanding of, let alone guarantee a conscientious response to, the ethical and moral problems science and technology can generate. Nor does scientific acumen impart special human or moral sensitivity. Yet that is what DTLM bureaucrats like Fauci often deceptively imply and expect us to believe.

As in war, facing a pandemic we must be extremely wary of conflicts of interests, particularly concealed profit and turf protection/expansion motives. *A pandemic is war by other means against an unexpected and utterly ruthless non-human enemy.* Nonetheless, it confronts us with challenges similar to ordinary wars, such as organizing resources, coordinating our tactics, and implementing a winning strategy, the same as we would do if we were battling a foreign military invasion. Deliberately hindering the efforts to combat a bio-threat can have the same effects as treason. War time profiteering can become a grave impediment to morale and the war effort itself, and so must be curbed.

The DTLM Complex in a pandemic is the equivalent of the military industrial complex in a standard war. With Covid, the Federal government, by default, allowed FDA procedures and DTLM profits to dictate our national strategy and tactics in three inappropriate and detrimental ways: 1) we prioritized only the weapons (vaccines) that would most profit the DTLM and rejected weapons (like ivermectin) that promised effectiveness but not huge profits; 2) aided by the tech giants, the DTLM pressured us to allow their commercial and professional ties with China to censor information, influence strategy, and handicap our efforts against Covid; 3) we allowed the DTLM to determine social, economic, and political policies that under the Constitution should be determined by elected officials.

In short, we allowed the DTLM Complex to run the war against Covid without adequate oversight from elected officials, and with inadequate input from critical stakeholders within society. It was rather like allowing defense contractors to launch a war on their own and then run it whatever ways they wanted, which would very likely be the ways most advantageous to themselves. In fact, critics accused the Bush Administration of doing just that during the Iraq war.

Who were the important but ignored stakeholders? —First and foremost were elderly patients vulnerable to Covid, then parents and their school age children, then doctors who actually treated Covid patients, people who own or work for small businesses, scientists and clinicians who disagreed with FDA, and people who want to practice their religion unencumbered by government interference. The biggest stakeholders were all those millions of American citizens who want to exercise their constitutionally guaranteed freedom to think about, discuss, and decide issues of great moment for the nation and then communicate their views to the rest of the citizenry without being hampered by politically motivated restrictions within what has displaced the press, post, and airwaves to become our prime medium of communication, the internet.

Perhaps most inexcusable is the travesty of the blue state public schools, emptied of their poor hapless, drifting, isolated, alienated children! Evidence from around the world continues to mount that school closures in a modern urbanized society, which were rarely medically justified during Covid, are in fact extremely damaging to all students from kindergarten to graduate school. There has been no significant difference between the youth Covid rates in states or countries that closed the schools compared to those who kept them open. The same goes for mandatory masking in schools. Thus, the claim that closures protect the children from Covid has been repeatedly debunked. One of the most definitive these efforts is from David Wallace-Wells:

> Over the course of the pandemic, 49,000 Americans under the age of 18 have died of all causes, according to the CDC. Only 331 of those deaths have been from COVID — less than half as many as have died of pneumonia. In 2019, more than 2,000 American kids and teenagers died in car crashes; each year

about a thousand die from drowning. More American children die in an average year from RSV — another respiratory ailment, whose prevalence is now growing because 18 months of quarantine have deprived young children of immune exposure — than died in either of the last two years from COVID-19.

Some of these comparisons aren't so neat, since the extraordinary precautions against COVID-19 prevented significant additional spread (and also suppressed the spread of other diseases). But, last year, fewer kids died of COVID-19 than of heart disease, "malignant neoplasms," suicide, and homicide — not to mention birth defects, which killed hundreds of times more. All told, 600,000 Americans have lost their lives to COVID over the course of the pandemic; just 0.05 percent of those were under the age of 18, a population that represents more than 20 percent of the country's population as a whole.[46]

It is truly shocking that so much of the US took the drastic step of closing schools for so long with so little consideration of negative consequences. Like "good Germans," we allowed teacher's union officials with hidden partisan agendas and deep conflicts of interest to simply lead us by the nose. Sweden and several other more sensible places, kept schools open, with no adverse consequences. Most US private and church schools remained open without significant Covid spread, as did most red state schools. However, the teachers' unions, which seem to think they own the Democrat party or at least believe they have hijacked it in league with the Wokesters, were often allowed in many states to dictate policy on school closures. Their injurious influence was profound in California, New York, Illinois, Washington, New Mexico, Nevada, New Jersey, Minnesota, Wisconsin, Michigan and other Democrat strongholds, especially in urban areas. Even where schools remained open students were often subject to masking requirements that were unhealthy and largely pointless in a school environment.

The Democrats of course are not the only party that allows special interests to dictate their public policies, witness the Republicans on abortion, contraception, and LGBT rights, or in respect to tax matters such as inheritance taxes, tax brackets, and loopholes like carried interest. Add to this the Republicans ignoring the routine predations against small investors by the financial industry and the massive unpunished financial fraud that led to TARP. But the unrelated sins of the GOP do not in any way excuse the Democrats bowing to the teachers' unions demands to close public schools.

The pure selfishness and irresponsibility of the union leaders is appalling. In order to protect the teachers from a miniscule and essentially theoretical medical risk, the school closures imposed on millions of children the risks of suicide, drug use, educational setbacks, and severe psychological sufferings from social isolation.[47] The closures also crippled the labor market and hobbled the entire economy by forcing parents, especially mothers, to stay off their jobs taking care of home bound children. The effect on millions of single moms who are disproportionately low income and minority has been devastating. America needs to realize that in our modern urbanized society we can no more shutter schools without dire consequences than we can stop collecting the garbage. Education is an essential service.

In the half of US schools that remained open there was no statistically significant evidence of students infecting teachers. But the teachers' unions didn't care about evidence, they closed the schools to gain advantages unrelated to Covid. Their teachers were paid full salary anyway and were free to find additional income in their ample spare time. The online learning was woefully inadequate, and it amplified the disadvantages of those students that were already behind. The social isolation crippled the students' psychological development. So, let's not mince words, the closure of the schools was criminally irresponsible and incredibly damaging to innocent children and youths as well as to the economies of states where closures prevailed. It is a truly shameful episode in our history. What a cynically irresponsible example to imprint upon a generation that will one day lead our nation!

New strains of Covid 19 are besieging us as I write this. We may well have another type of Corona or other viral pandemic in the near future. We cannot again allow schools closures simply because Woke teachers' union officials want to hold our children hostage as a bargaining chip for a union agenda unrelated to the health crisis we all face. President Reagan fired the striking air traffic controllers; similar draconic measures against the teachers' unions, such as cut offs of federal funding were fully justified, but never taken, during Covid. President Trump may have wanted to act like Reagan, but already the most vilified President since Lincoln, Trump must have been wary of further retribution from the Trump Derangement Democrats and their media allies, not to mention sabotage and back stabbing from Dr. Fauci, FDA, and the DTLM complex.

The total US efforts against Covid were disastrously chaotic and uncoordinated, as you might expect with each state pursuing its own policies. Instead of decisive national leadership we had leadership from state governors that at times seemed headed in fifty different directions. Not since the Civil War has America been so fractured and divided against itself. With the next pandemic we will have less excuse for lack of coordination and political factions going for each other's throats. Imagine if the US were at war with another country, say Germany or Japan in World War II, and we left coordination of war efforts up to the states, with the Federal government offering only non-binding recommendations. What if you had some states going all out, others holding back, some refusing to do anything, and with no overall coordination of either strategy or tactics?

Well, some wars are fought that way, and they are almost always lost that way. Generally speaking, we lost the war against Covid insofar as our chaotic cross purposes inflicted far more suffering and collateral damage to the economy and the health and sanity of our people and society than was needed to contain and manage the virus. Worst of all, our struggle with Corvid and related viral pandemics is not over, it may be that it has only just begun.

Chapter 7

Six Rules for Doing Better Next Time.

Laws are like cobwebs, which may catch small flies,
but let wasps and hornets break through.
— Jonathan Swift

1. **FIRST, ETERNAL VIGILANCE:** Realize that, for the foreseeable future, bureaucracy, like bad weather, poverty, crime, and fatal illnesses, will remain an unavoidable and ubiquitous problem. So we must be ever on guard against bureaucratic abuses. We must respect, protect, and reward whistleblowers, and devise improved oversight on and accountability for all bureaucracies, governmental, corporate, and non-profit. The public needs to understand that bureaucracies and bureaucrats going rogue are the greatest systematic threat to democracy and our personal freedoms. Totalitarianism begins when the bureaucracies go rogue, or are beholden to a single party and its elite.

2. **TERM LIMITS FOR BUREAUCRATS as well as for politicians.** Many thanks to Dr. Anthony S. Fauci for doing such a brilliant job alerting us to this crying need/urgent problem. It makes sense to limit terms for all powerful officials, whether elected or appointed, to a generation which runs twenty to twenty-four years. Limiting those who hold powerful positions to a generation follows the natural order. Allowing individual bureaucrats to control critical positions for more than a generation creates impediments to social, political, economic, and technological adaptation to the challenges of a changing world. Once in power, bureaucrats, politicians etc., rarely forsake the ways of thinking and acting that brought them to power. Often, the only effective way to adapt institutions to historic changes is to change personnel.

Some might object that a standard cut off after 20 years backed by a mandatory limit of 24 years would not make much difference because officials seldom hold their positions that long. Nevertheless, knowing there is a time limit can impact the way bureaucrats regard themselves and their jobs by curbing their tendency to conflate professional *personae* with who they are, that is with their real identities. We need to shift the bureaucrats' self-identification from "I am Governor" to "I serve(d) as Governor." To promote policy flexibility and innovation, we must change how the bureaucrats see their positions in the bureaucracy—that must be as temporary and provisional, never inviolable and inalienable as it is in a monarchy or in a credentialed "scientific" elite. Assuming an identity for life may work well for the current Queen of England who is a unique, beloved, and widely respected figure, but it's counterproductive for officials running any governmental, corporate, or non-profit bureaucracy.[48]

3. **SUNSET EVERY PROGRAM, RE-EVALUATE EVERY POLICY PERIODICALLY.** Every government institution, agency, policy, and procedure needs to be re-assessed and re-evaluated periodically on a cost/effectiveness and risk/benefit basis. Successful businesses do this routinely, so should government bureaucracies. Regrettably, it doesn't happen at FDA, NIH, CDC, or Dr. Fauci's NIAID. We will never want to eliminate the police, garbage collection, or firemen (lessons from Chicago, Portland, Minneapolis et al.), but every job and function within those departments needs regular up-dating and periodic re-invention. Nowhere is this more necessary than in healthcare and in education.

Berkshire-Hathaway may provide a useful paradigm for government bureaucracies in its annual re-evaluations of all areas of its businesses. Do not the American people deserve an annual report on all aspects of their government as thorough and thoughtful as the ones Warren Buffett provides his investors? Perhaps Warren should have run for President on a platform to enact a program of continuous re-evaluation of the Federal bureaucracy to promote its efficiency and insure accountability! It might have been a prudent investment of his time with superb returns for his investors and for all Americans.

4. RESTRICT REVOLVING DOOR TRANSFERS FROM GOVERNMENT TO BUSINESSES, LIMIT AND ROUTINELY SCRUTINIZE OUTSIDE CONSULTANT GIGS. Revolving doors can create closed, incestuous societies where new ideas and new people are unwelcome and a CYA attitude prevails. Promotion becomes a matter of who you know, not what you can do. Again Dr. Fauci's realm of the DTLM complex, especially the FDA, provides countless examples of the inefficiencies and the damage wrought by the revolving door.

5. **CREATE MORE EFFECTIVE SYSTEMS OF OVERSIGHT, ACCOUNTABILITY, AND ENFORCEMENT FOR BUREAUCRACIES.** Through their guiding principle of checks and balances, the Founding Fathers sought to establish competing levels of government accountability that would safeguard the freedoms of individual citizens and curb undue accumulations of power among government officials. With the explosion of bureaucracy in the 20th century, e.g., DOJ, DOD, IRS, CIA, DEA, FBI, FDA, NIH, NIAID, CDC, these agencies, led by their grand avatars J. Edgar Hoover and Anthony S. Fauci, have evolved rigorous systems of internal surveillance and enforcement designed to keep employees in line, limit free expression and creative thought within their fiefdoms, shape public perception, minimize outside oversight, and eliminate accountability. No whistleblowers dare act where J. Edgar and Tony Fauci reign! Despite the abundance of complaints about and evidence for FBI abuses arising from partisan bias, not a single FBI whistleblower has dared to step forward to call out specific abuses of power under Robert, Mueller, James Comey, and Christopher Wray. Why do you think that is? What are potential whistle blowers afraid of?

Generally speaking, neither Congress, nor the media, nor the public yet recognize the magnitude of the threat to democracy and personal rights our giant rogue, overlord bureaucracies pose. Few realize that a criminal bureaucracy is far more dangerous and destructive than any individual criminal can be. To counter these threats, we would need to institute an additional system of checks and balances for improved oversight on government agencies and their bureaucracies. Checks and balances among the three branches of government keep these branches in line in respect to each other much of the time. However, the current limited system has proved to be a woefully unreliable and insufficient brake on the excesses of rogue Federal bureaucracies and bureaucrats. Although these bureaucracies are parts of the executive branch, in many cases the President exercises scant control and they habitually ignore or even defy directives from the White House, serving instead their unelected officials own partisan ends. Just as bad, they sometimes illegally serve the President's partisan objectives, as when the IRS or the FBI harass or target a President's political opponents. In either case they are going rogue and ours is no longer a government of laws.

Exiting the Constitutional Convention in 1787, Benjamin Franklin was asked what kind of government they had given us. Franklin famously replied, "a Republic if you can keep it." Balance of power under the principle of checks and balances is the main constitutional reason we have been able to keep Franklin's Republic so long. However, the Constitutional Convention took place decades before big government with its proliferation of independent agencies and bureaucracies led by increasingly arrogant and wayward bureaucracies began to develop. Today we sorely lack effective checks and balances on our proliferation of powerful, autonomous federal agencies, the overlords of the Swamp. Where in our system can you find effective oversight on the FBI, the CIA, the DEA, DOJ, IRS, FDA, CDC, NIH, or the august Dr./St. Fauci? Who was watching Fauci when he diverted NIH funds into gain of function research in Wuhan China?

The very idea of oversight on the great bureaucracies and their leaders provokes smiles among those familiar with the ways of the Swamp. The occasional congressional hearing or letter, or Inspector General report almost never changes anything. President Trump had close to zero effective oversight on his intransigent DOJ and rogue FBI, even though the Constitution made him their legitimate boss. A big part of Trump's problem was bad initial appointments. If he had made Rudi Giuliani or perhaps Chris Christie his first AG, the history of Trump's presidency would have been very different. Agencies that ignore the officials elected by the people to oversee them are no longer accountable to the people, period. That makes them very dangerous to our democracy and a threat to our precious personal freedoms.

America needs to wake up! Federal bureaucracies can too easily become rogue actors, as the FBI and CIA occasionally have been throughout much of their histories and the FDA has frequently been since the 1962 Kefauver-Harris FDA Amendment. When that happens, there is little to stop bureaucracies from brushing aside the interests of the public, ignoring elected officials, and trampling on the rights of individual citizens. A Senator Rand Paul deserves respect because he was elected by the people who deserve respect. No voters ever elected or had a chance to vote out of office Anthony Fauci, Stephen Hahn, James Comey, or Christopher Wray. Like Henry VIII and Louis XIV, they act as if they assume they were elevated into their positions by God. In Fauci's case it's the great god of modernity, Science, who has another identity in his ruling Faustus myth.

Independent ombudsmen style courts might constitute an effective step in the direction of better oversight, but they would require far greater independence and enforcement powers than agency Inspector General officials currently possess. A special system of oversight courts is needed to process public or citizen complaints and charges against bureaucracies and powerful bureaucrats. It could in some respects be modeled on and take inspiration from Nelson Mandela's concept of Truth and Reconciliation. We need to make it easier for individual citizens to file complaints and bring charges against unreasonable or dysfunctional bureaucratic policies, practices, directives, and regulations, as well as against individual bureaucrats and bureaucracies that function in ways that are unjust, ineffectual, or violate individual rights and the principles of democracy.

Instituting the new oversight courts might require a Constitutional amendment, which is likely needed anyway to address the array of problems created by the vast new fourth branch of government that the writers of the constitution failed to anticipate—I refer, of course, to the increasingly autonomous three letter overlord agencies whose bureaucracies did not begin to emerge until a century after the Constitutional convention. These, much more than Congress, the President or the Federal courts have become the Big Brother face our government shows to the average American citizen.

The new oversight courts should be empowered to impose reparations and give recommendations to Congress or the President for correcting systemic injustices that stem from bureaucratic abuses or culpable inefficiencies. In our day, systemic injustices have become an almost radioactive issue. Among the younger generation there is growing demand to correct long standing systemic injustices in the area of race. But why limit long standing injustices to racial matters? All injustice is morally wrong, psychologically damaging, and socially deleterious. With characteristic expediency, the left has shifted Marx's focus on class injustices to racial injustices: either focus is much too limiting. We need to find ways to root out and rectify injustices wherever they occur. This must include the injustices of bureaucracies to specific individuals, not just to groups. Here is a truth we should never forget: ***Groups are not capable of suffering injustices, only the individuals within groups suffer, and always in varying degrees.*** Thinking that ethics are about groups is the Marxist way, but it is not the American way and it deviates from the Judeo-Christian ethic's prime focus on the rights, sufferings, and free choices of responsible individuals.

6. DEVELOP RISK EVALUATION STANDARDS AND PROCEDURES. TEACH ALL AMERICANS TO WEIGH RISK CAREFULLY, AND PRIORITIZE RISKS IN ALL AREAS OF LIFE ACCORDING TO THEIR LEVELS OF PROBABILITY AS WELL AS DEGREES OF PERIL. BE EVER WARY OF BUREAUCRATS, GOVERNMENTAL AND OTHER, WHO INCITE RISK HYSTERIA TO INCREASE THEIR POWER, FUNDING, AND PROFITS. Risk evaluation should be taught in schools along with civics, another vital subject that has been largely ignored or perverted in recent years. The history of the FDA, CIA, NIH, DOJ, CDC, IRS, and FBI provide countless examples of the desperate need for this reform. Inciting risk hysteria (shouting fire in a crowded theater) is harmful, and when done for gain it is criminal. We need laws enforced with strict penalties whose purpose is to expose and counter bureaucratic promotion and exploitation of risk hysteria.

Chapter 8

What to Do About The FDA?

Ecrasez l' enfame
— Voltaire on the Church

To protect Constitutional government along with citizen rights, reform is needed in varying degrees with all of our three-letter swamp overlords who grow ever more powerful and are seldom accountable to anyone but themselves. Certainly, they are insufficiently accountable to either their titular boss, the President of the United States, or to Congress. Rarely do the courts end up vindicating the people against the FDA which can spend unlimited amounts of tax money fighting court challenges from individual citizens who have scant resources. With FDA the need for fundamental change is especially urgent because that agency's mistakes and abuses can be exceptionally costly in human lives. However, these abuses are difficult to document for three main reasons: 1) they often involve arcane scientific disputes where consensus is lacking or where courts are reluctant to venture; 2) FDA's powers of retribution against its critics along with its ability to pick the winners and losers in its drug approval lottery; 3) and the flaws of FDA's institutional culture are so engrained, convoluted, and deep seated.

If further research and investigation confirm conclusively that ivermectin, hydroxychloroquine, and other Covid treatment and prevention alternatives gratuitously trashed by FDA might have saved tens thousands of lives the agency itself must be held strictly accountable. Holding it accountable, nonetheless, will be extraordinarily difficult because of FDA's vast power as chief overlord within the DTLM Complex. Doctors and researchers who try to hold the agency accountable typically suffer retribution and professional ostracism; publically criticizing FDA is definitely not a wise career move for anyone working in the areas FDA regulates. Yet to fail to hold FDA accountable would be a criminally irresponsible betrayal of the American people on the part of Congress and the President who have legal oversight on FDA, however rarely and ineffectively they exercise that oversight.

I fear that betrayal will very likely happen---'cover up and forget' is how the Swamp and our irresponsible political class likes to resolve their own crimes and scandals. Every sign indicates that the Swamp is expanding and its partisan corruption grows ever deeper in the current political chaos. The FDA is a monster born in and bred for the swamp, so expect the Swamp to defend its own.

But what if FDA is correct, that all the alternative treatments like ivermectin will be found to lack significant efficacy in scientific trials not run by FDA or by people under its retributory influence, but in honest, objective trials nearly everyone accepts as valid? In my experience, during the US AIDS epidemic in the late 1980s until 1996, many alternative treatments were tried and also hyped, sometimes shamelessly. A few doctors who appeared to be reputable claimed to be getting "interesting" results. A few patients like Ron Woodruff of the Dallas Buyer's Club claimed this or that treatment was working for them. Martin Delaney, Tony Fauci's best friend in AIDS activism, hyped a Chinese abortifacient he called Compound Q and managed to persuade a few hundred patients to try it in the year or two before it fizzled. However, among all these desperate attempts we never saw efficacy claims and evidence remotely comparable to what we've seen with ivermectin and hydroxychloroquine.

Studies with thousands of patients made by substantial numbers of reputable clinicians in India, Mexico, Peru and around the world claim safety and efficacy for these two drugs. Moreover, large numbers of doctors across the US are prescribing them with what they insist are excellent results. I've checked back months later with doctors who had told me they prescribe them. Not one of these doctors reported that they stopped prescribing the drugs because they found that they really did not work or had serious safety issues. It's anecdotal I know, but how likely is it that all these doctors are deluded fools or liars conspiring to put one over on the world and their profession? If so, that would be a scam and/or conspiracy of unprecedented magnitude. It would be quite difficult to explain considering that these far flung doctors do not know each other or even speak the same native tongue, and they gain nothing but the joy of seeing their patients recover. For helping their patients stay alive, they risk fierce blowback from the DTLM Complex, the FDA, and government officials as well as from big tech and the Woke cancel culture. Given the problematic history of the DTLM Complex and the FDA it is easier to believe they are the real conspirators trying to bury a treatment that they don't own and control than it is to believe that all these unconnected family physicians across the globe have somehow set up a vast conspiracy that gains them nothing. FDA was habitually dishonest and unscrupulous during the AIDS epidemic: a leopard does not change its spots.

But just for the sake of argument, let us say that FDA is proven right to my satisfaction and even Fox News, Mark Levin, Harvey Risch, Bret Weinstein, Pierre Cory et al agree that these drugs are essentially placebos. There still would be plenty of other compelling reasons why FDA should have been reformed, re-organized, and re-invented decades ago. The case for radical change at FDA does not depend on proving the agency played a destructive role in the Covid pandemic, though I am convinced that it did and continues to do so. FDA, along with the entire DTLM complex, needs reform beyond reform to speed medical innovation and reduce healthcare costs. Irrespective of the merits of the cases for ivermectin etc., the evidence is overwhelming that FDA needlessly delays overall medical innovation, and its regulatory over-kill drives up US medical costs far higher than in similar advanced countries like Canada, UK, France, Japan, Taiwan, Germany, Australia, Sweden, Denmark, and even Switzerland.

Here is the prime lesson from the recent history of FDA, as well as other 3 letter overlords like the NIH and the FBI: *We need to apply trust bust thinking to governmental entities—something that's rarely been done before but should be started ASAP.* We need to break up many of the Swamp overlord agencies the way Teddy Roosevelt did with the monopolistic industrial trusts. The most urgent place to begin is the agency at the heart of the DTLM Complex trust, the US Food and Drug Administration. Of course, we must retain the current functions of FDA whose purpose is to insure the safety of our food, pharmaceuticals, and other medical supplies. However, these functions should be placed under separate administrative structures. The current FDA umbrella creates needless layers of bureaucracy that only slow innovation and generate waste and corruption.

Food could and should be transferred out of FDA along with diagnostic tests and medical devices. Regulation in many areas, especially food and devices, might be better done by non-government entities, such as Underwriters Laboratories does with electrical devices, or farmed out the way FAA does with its evaluations of new commercial aircraft. Rarely is government the most efficient way of doing anything. Biotech, nanotech, gene therapy, and other frontier technologies could be better handled by an agency separate from that dealing with standard pharmaceuticals. The issues, technical expertise, and outlook necessary in these areas is often quite different from that needed in pharmaceuticals. With new, rapidly advancing technologies, smaller, more independent, resilient, and nimble regulatory bodies are more likely to promote creativity and innovation. Nothing is gained and much could be potentially lost by keeping the regulation of new technologies at the frontier of medical innovation under the thumb of the ossified FDA behemoth.

Currently, FDA's reflex reaction to nearly every new medical and healthcare innovation is to delay approval with extensive, protracted fine tuning of testing the degrees of efficacy. However, once safety is established, the most meaningful places to determine degrees of efficacy become the clinic and the marketplace. The risk averse culture of FDA founded on its sacrosanct thalidomide narrative of a heroic (on leave) Dr. Francis Kelsey saving the American public from the horrors of hideously deformed babies through delayed drug approval, well it is fairy tale.[49] Sorry, FDA but your fairy tale leaves out uncomfortable facts and is belied by the opposing true stories of your (fortunately) thwarted attempts to delay the AIDS cocktails, and your repeated delays on too many other valuable treatments for cancer and other killers.[50] By using their thalidomide myth to justify pushing to the limits regulations enacted under the 1962 FDA Kefauver-Harris Amendment, FDA vastly expanded its power to delay or even thwart drug approvals. The Amendment allowed the agency to extend efficacy testing to a cripplingly convoluted level. Thereby, FDA gained the power to play God by picking the winners and losers, the wet dream of evil bureaucrats everywhere.[51]

Mary Ruwart has detailed in *Death by Regulation*, FDA's expansion of regulation under the 1962 FDA Amendment. The Amendment, Ruwart concludes have failed the test of cost effectiveness:

> *Dr. Dale Gieringer of Stanford University estimated that without the Amendments 5000-10,000 US lives would have been lost had the FDA approved the same drugs that the Britain had. However, Americans would have gotten lifesaving drugs earlier without the Amendments, thus saving 21,000 to 120,000 lives. In other words, Gieringer found that the delays in approvals were more deadly than the extra side effects that came from a more rapid approval process.[52]*

FDA would likely counter that Gieringer and Ruwart need much more rigorous and thorough studies to make their case. Well, why don't we have them? Why has the Federal government failed to conduct thorough, objective *outside studies* to determine whether the 1962 Amendment actually benefits the American people? At least three obstacles stand in the way: first, FDA would oppose such studies and lobby against them with Congress, the White House and the general public; second, if Congress authorized them, FDA would want to conduct them and thereby slow and slant the results; third, the Federal government does not normally commission such independent oversight reviews of government agencies, which is one reason why there is so much waste in Washington.

And so FDA continues to demagogically push their Thalidomide fairy tale with its dishonest risk hysteria in order to rationalize prolonged testing of something quite different, drug efficacy. Testing safety gives FDA limited power because drugs are normally either safe within the parameters of their specified uses, or they are too unsafe to be approved. Efficacy testing allows FDA a far wider range of discretion, and far greater ability to manipulate, shape, expand, and restrict the market for a drug. FDA has never published a clear definition of its efficacy standard, so there is no scientific way to determine if any particular drug meets that standard. We don't even know if FDA has ever formulated an efficacy standard, though they were required to do so by Congress. Instead of a specific efficacy standard, FDA has advisory panels, but its ultimately up to the FDA bureaucrats, not the panels, to decide.

We saw this play out disturbingly in the agency's recent controversial approval of Biogen's adulcanumab, a monoclonal antibody with the brand name Aduhelm, for treating early stage Alzheimer's disease. The approval was highly controversial because FDA over-ruled its advisory panel's recommendation against approval. The panel determined that the drug made no statistically significant improvements in the patients' mental abilities. Other critics lambasted the drug's $56,000/year cost as outrageous for a drug that lacks demonstrated efficacy. What Aduhelm did demonstrate, once again, was that in practice FDA uses the efficacy standard and the 1962 Amendment as a virtual carte blanche allowing the agency to do whatever it pleases. Perhaps the Gates Foundation could do something constructive and run parallel efficacy trials testing the $56,000.00 adulcanumab in early stage Alzheimer's against a $35.00 course of ivermectin with early stage Covid 19. We might learn a lot about how FDA's undefined efficacy standard works in practice, and why it should be challenged.

FDA expands its power by trying or at least pretending to measure the degree of efficacy, not just the fact of efficacy. However, evidence for the fact of efficacy is the only reasonable requirement for drug approval. The degree of efficacy always varies with multiple factors such as dosage, age, weight, sex, and race of patients, other drugs used, the patient's other diseases, and his/her unique genetic makeup, and specific personal circumstances. That means the most reliable and important place to test drug efficacy is in the clinics and in the medical/healthcare marketplace. Adulcanumab failed on both the fact and degree of efficacy, according to FDA's own expert panel. *(Something for New York Post's Miranda Divine to look into: did Biogen retain any FDA consultants named Hunter?)*

A reformed FDA must shift the burden of drug evaluation from pre-market efficacy testing to post market efficacy and safety monitoring. Most actual adverse drug with drug effects, along with the finer details of efficacy, are discovered after drugs are released into the market and are in wide use in 'imperfect' patients on other medications. By testing degrees of efficacy in extravagant randomized placebo controlled pre-market trials, FDA gains something new that Congress did not intend to give them---power to influence and even control the marketability of a drug along with the marketing, and ultimately the profits, of private companies. With the rise of the DTLM complex and big pharma, FDA's power to control the drug market became power to control vast wealth---and controlling the money is what it's all about within the DTLM complex.

One alternative to the current FDA that could expedite innovation and empower patients would be to establish a two track system of drug, device, and biotech approval. A streamlined version of current FDA procedures would be retained to give drugs full approval including estimating the degrees of efficacy, which on large scale medical conditions, like arthritis, can be useful for private insurance, Medicare, and Medicaid purposes. Such "full approval" could be supplemented by post-market monitoring of safety and efficacy. A secondary tract would first test safety and then test to determine the fact, though not the degree, of efficacy. It would be authorized to give accelerated approval on the basis of safety and basic evidence for the fact of efficacy. Patients, in consultation with their doctors, would then be free to try safety tested new drugs much earlier in their development process. The accelerated tract would need to be independent of the regular FDA, possibly with a private group. Having a second track would give patients with life threatening conditions more options, the so far largely imperfectly realized intent of Congress in passing the 'right to try' legislation which eases but does not end FDA obstruction. It would also give the parent FDA competition that could help speed, refine, and improve its work. As a rule, competition is healthy, and FDA's history shows that the agency could really benefit from some effective, independent competition.

If it becomes indisputable that by covertly as well as overtly sabotaging the use of ivermectin, hydroxychloroquine etc., as prevention and treatment of Covid, FDA, Fauci, and their DTLM colluders and co-conspirators blocked the use of drugs or supplements that, if promptly and widely deployed, could have saved tens maybe even hundreds of thousands of American lives, it will become imperative that Congress the President act to prevent recurrence. Intentionally, or more likely instinctually, the DTLM Complex may well have greatly amplified the

Covid disaster in America in order to increase the vaccine profits of the DTLM companies and just to maintain and expand their power and turf. Whether or not they are guilty of blocking valuable Covid treatments, FDA, Fauci, and the DTLM must not be allowed to continue their practice of setting the rules of the game so that they get to pick the winners and losers in medical innovation.

The American people need and deserve the full truth about the entire Covid crisis, particularly the true roles and the details on the behind the scenes actions of China, Dr. Fauci, FDA, and others in the DTLM Complex. In an ideal world when the whole truth is out, blame and credit should be assessed so that appropriate reforms and prosecutions can follow. The whole truth and nothing but the truth is usually necessary for effective reforms to be enacted and always necessary for justice to prevail. King Lear's fool tells us what's more likely in the real world of the DC Swamp--denial, cover up, and continued malfeasance:

> *Truth's a dog must to kennel; he must be whipped out'/When*
> *Lady the brach may stand by the fire and stink. (I. iv. 66-7.*

Blocking the alternative drugs for Covid treatment was medically inexcusable since they were clearly safe having been used by millions for decades. Here's the rub, FDA, Fauci and the DTLM went beyond their mandates by interfering in the prescription by doctors and use by patients of long approved, clearly safe drugs. This is really a market issue where the judgment of clinical professionals and the feedback from the patients ought to be the final regulator. FDA and Fauci and other DTLM players, who thrive on monopolies, have never been satisfied with leaving anything to the free market, especially not the free market in ideas. On the last point, they enjoy fierce, unrelenting support from the tech giants and the Woke cancel culture.

The DTLM interference was worse than just inexcusable, it was likely criminal in a moral if not a specifically US legal sense. The individuals responsible should be investigated and punished if found guilty of damaging patients or deceiving the public. The institutions responsible, the FDA along with NIAID, CDC and their accomplices in the DTLM Complex, must all be radically reformed if their malfeasance is found to have cost America countless lives and trillions of its wealth.

We need to do this in order to send a clear message to other rogue actors among our three letter Swamp overlords. Otherwise, we have no protection against similar misconduct and wrongdoing being repeated in future health emergencies and spreading across the board throughout the Swamp and into all areas of American life.

Indeed, the past conduct of Dr. Fauci, FDA, and the DTLM gives us every reason to believe they will go on doing whatever profits and empowers them most until we stop them. As I said before, my *How FDA Challenged America and Saved FDA from Itself* details the FDA's attempts to delay the HIV drug cocktails that transformed AIDS from a death sentence to a manageable disease. Had not their plans been thwarted by an alliance of activists and patients backed by their conscientious doctors and researchers, tens of thousands of additional AIDS sufferers would have died waiting three additional years for FDA to pace through its cumbersome formalities with additional efficacy tests on what we already knew were life-saving drugs. Yet FDA was never called into account, and so nothing that was wrong has been changed.

History repeats itself, unless we recognize our mistakes and correct them. We cannot predict when the next pandemic will strike, where it will come from, or how severe it will be any more than we predicted Covid 19. The AIDS pandemic killed considerably more than has Covid, and these were mostly younger people in the prime of their lives: the number of years of life lost to AIDS was exponentially greater than the number lost to Covid. Pandemics come suddenly and take the populace unawares. Quick action is always urgent, and quick action is clearly not FDA's forte. Our survival may depend on having organizational structures far better tailored to rapid response with pandemics and to accelerating medical innovation in general.

FDA has shown with AIDS and with Covid that its self-protective behavior, methods, and culture, especially its resort to risk hysteria in place of balanced risk evaluation, will also cause needless, unjustifiable delays in getting out viable treatments for pandemics. If America and its divisive, self-serving politicians fail to reform the FDA, the American people may well be left defenseless against the next pandemic. We may die unnecessarily by the hundreds of thousands, or worse millions, because

FDA bars or impedes access to and approval of treatments that can save many of the afflicted. Meanwhile, patients will again be made to wait for FDA and the DTLM to manipulate and approve treatments or vaccines in accordance with their profit, power, turf, and political agendas. The choice for America is stark and unequivocal. We must dismantle the current FDA and reform its functions to establish better oversight on and accountability for the DTLM Complex. Otherwise far too many people will suffer and die needlessly in the next pandemic.

Congress must start the reform process by repealing the 1962 FDA Amendment and replacing it with unmistakable guidelines for FDA's, or better yet its successor agencies,' new mission: protecting, promoting, and facilitating medical innovation. The next Republican President, or Democrat President if we should be so fortunate as to get one who is able and inclined to take on FDA, must appoint a new FDA commissioner with clear, well thought out FDA reform plans. A crucial step must be re-education. The FDA's successor agencies need to cleanse the "risk averse culture" of the past with training courses teaching their personnel to recognize and reject risk hysteria. Instead, they must learn to evaluate relative risk within the broad context of risk filled human life. This should include fully exposing the Thalidomide myth for the deceptive fairy tale it is. They must also teach all FDA employees the full, unvarnished truth about FDA's obstructive actions in the "COVID crisis" as well as about FDA's deadly past delays in approving cancer and AIDS medicines, including their failed attempt to delay approval of the AIDS drug cocktails. To avoid repeating FDA's past mistakes, FDA's successors must fully acknowledge, understand, and repudiate them.

Epilogue

Civilizations die from suicide, not by murder.
— *Arnold Toynbee*

Will humanity and human civilization survive? Will humanity annihilate itself and join the vast horde of magnificent species that we heedless humans have driven to extinction? History shows that the things we feared most are seldom the threats that pose our greatest dangers. None of the ancient empires fell the ways their leaders and peoples most feared they would. Few anticipated that mighty Persia would face total defeat and conquest at the hands of Alexander of Macedon. The Byzantines did not foresee the coming of Mohammad and his armies. The fourteenth century Europeans did not expect the black plague to decimate their populations and set in motion a Renaissance that brought changes such as the world had never seen before. Who foresaw the rise of science, Copernicus, Galileo, Newton, Darwin, and Einstein, the rebirth of the arts to unprecedented glory, or the revolution in psychology with Freud and Jung? Who expected an English villager improbably named Shakespeare would write more great plays than all those written by all playwrights before and after him, and make the English language a uniquely potent force in spreading Western civilization across the entire globe? Shakespeare would have marveled at our cinema, but even he would not have imagined it. And not just Shakespeare stands out, who expected Michelangelo, Leonardo, Velasquez, Cervantes, Milton, Voltaire, Bach, Mozart, Beethoven, and Tolstoy? —each a miracle without precedent.

In early 1914 none expected the most terrible war ever would soon rage across Europe and destroy the centuries old Russian, German, Austrian, and Turkish empires. The US founding fathers did not believe their union would shatter over slavery, and they never imagined that less than four score years after its nation rending Civil War America would become the greatest power the world had ever seen, spearheading the spread of democratic ideals and institutions across the globe. Abraham Lincoln would not have imagined that the nation he had saved from dissolution would develop the hydrogen bomb or send men to the moon one hundred and four years after his death. In 1984 few imagined the Soviet Union would fall a mere seven years hence or foresaw the meteoric rises of China, Islamic Jihad, and American Marxism, let alone the internet. I foresaw the rise of China, but not the other trends. The big events we fear or hope for usually do not happen. More often we are surprised by the totally unexpected appearing, it seems, from nowhere.

If history teaches us anything certain, it is that mankind has never learned to govern itself. The current Covid chaos shows how dire our deficiencies of government leadership are. Our current leaders are unremarkable; they appear to have learned nothing from history. Despite our vast populations to draw from, we have no one remotely in the same league as Cyrus, Pericles, Caesar, Elizabeth I, Washington, Napoleon, or Lincoln. Furthermore, Hitler, Stalin, and Mao were more destructive leaders of great, highly civilized nations than any before their times. This trend may warn of worse to come.

Nonetheless, I believe civilization does have a chance to survive, if somehow we can find better ways to govern ourselves. The biggest threats may not be climate change, asteroid strikes, plagues, wars, or depletion of resources—science and technology are capable of finding ways to disarm them all. My nominee would be bureaucracy. Hitler, Stalin, and Mao showed us how readily bureaucracies and bureaucrats embrace evil, and what a weak brake the ethics of individual citizens are against a powerful, malign bureaucracy, especially bureaucracies controlled by sociopaths.

Bureaucracy almost turned the whole of Germany into a nation of Adolf Eichmanns who were "only following orders," and Eichmann had his multiple Russian and Chinese counterparts. Most educated people recognize this fact. What we fail to recognize is a truth much harder to accept: Eichmann has his American, British, French, Japanese, Mexican, Indian, Iranian, Israeli, Nigerian, and even Swiss and Norwegian counterparts lodged in our bureaucracies. Covid 19 should have demonstrated this, but so far its lessons have not taken hold. My readers, I suspect, can think of some prominent Covid era candidates for Adolf Eichmann's dark role.

So will civilization survive? To survive we must first recognize ***humanity's biggest challenge: governing ourselves***. All modern systems of government depend on bureaucracy and we do not know how to exercise effective oversight on bureaucracy let alone enforce accountability on bureaucrats. Humanity's one real advance in government has been democracy which, when it works well, allows the people to exercise oversight on and even replace the government itself, but the people remain stuck with the bureaucracies. Churchill said that democracy is the worst form of government, except all the others. One of democracy's main strengths lies in its ability to improve oversight on bureaucracy. But the bureaucracies always resist oversight and accountability from the people or their elected representatives who with good reason distrust the motives and fear the power of the bureaucrats.

America with its constitutional democracy found ways to give the people limited power over elected officials. However, the writers of the Constitution did not anticipate the rise of our massive, opaque bureaucracies with vast treasuries to spend and armies of bureaucrats to deploy and command. And so they failed to give either the people or their elected representatives effective instruments for oversight on discipline of today's huge, immensely powerful, self-contained and potentially very dangerous bureaucracies. Moreover, the bureaucrats have earned how to sidestep, sideline, and ignore the people and their elected representatives.

The people assume that the task of the bureaucrats is to solve their problems, and most people presume, naively, that the bureaucrats will act in good faith. Why should they when their own interests conflict with those of the people? Why not serve their own interests if there is no effective oversight on them, if the people have no ways to make them accountable? Look at FDA, CIA, and FBI, when have these great American overlords been made accountable? History shows that without oversight and accountability, bureaucrats will either ignore the people's problems or address them by only those means that further the bureaucrats own interests.

The sum and substance is this: first we must recognize that bureaucrats without effective oversight and accountability can never just be trusted to act in the interests of the people or relied on to faithfully do what the people's democratically elected representatives tell them. Thus, the survival of democracy and civilization itself will require establishing far more effective oversight on and accountability for bureaucrats within our most powerful bureaucracies. In these challenges America, the world's leading democracy, is failing miserably. Bureaucratic evil has many faces, but the one face that most often draws mankind into the abyss of destruction is not that of a Hitler, or Stalin, or Mao, or Pol Pot, but of Adolf Eichmann, the innocuous seeming, by the book, banal bureaucrat who only did what he was told.

End Notes

1. Cabot, Katy, *Jung, My Mother and I*, (Infidel, Switz: Daimon Verlag, 2001) p.322.
2. "U.S. Life Expectancy fell by a year in the first half of 2020, CDC reports," *Stat, 2/18/21.*
3. Deace, Steve & Erzen, Todd, *A Faucian Bargain*, (New York: Post Hill Press, 2021) p. 69.
4. See: "Lockdowns Have Protected the Rich at the Expense of Working Class People," Lucy Johnston, *Express* UK, July 2, 2021. Johnson provides an extended discussion of the reasons non lockdown states have done better than heavy lockdown states during Covid. She focuses on Florida, but her observations apply to similar situations across the US and the world. Outside of Asia, Sweden's next door neighbors, Norway and Denmark, are among the very few places where lockdowns worked well, but at a much higher economic price than Sweden paid. Strict lockdowns appeared to be working well in Thailand at first, but today they are getting around 20,000 cases per day, about the same as the US or Mexico but among a much smaller population. People in Thailand are blaming the "crappy" Chinese vaccine used there. So far, the "science" on the lockdowns is inconclusive. They appear to work some places some of the time, but not in all places and not even in different places at different times. Information on how lockdowns were conducted and how well they worked in China would be very useful. Unfortunately, the CCP is not obliging here.
5. Technically, it would have been complex though possible for Donald Trump to fire Fauci, who was not appointed by the President but by the head of NIH. Trump would have needed to choose an NIH chief committed to Fauci's near term retirement; that would have been possible, Mike Pence's likely opposition notwithstanding.
6. C-Span transcript of Oct. 4, 1988 Pres. Debate.
7. Kolata, Gina, NYT, Mar 26, 1990, *Radical Change Urged in Testing of AIDS Drugs.*
8. Nussbaum, Bruce, *Good Intentions* (New York: The Atlantic Monthly Press, 1990) pp 136-149.
9. Driscoll, James, *How AIDS Activists Challenged America* (Washington-London: Academica Press, 2020) p 144.
10. Andrzejewsky, Adam, "Dr. Anthony Fauci: The Highest Paid Employee in the Entire US Federal Government," (*Forbes,* Jan 25,2021) "Dr. Anthony Fauci made $417,608 in 2019, the latest year for which federal salaries are available. That made him not only the highest paid doctor in the federal

government, but the highest paid out of all four million federal employees. In fact, Dr. Fauci even made more than the $400,000 salary of the President of the United States. All salary data was collected by OpenTheBooks.com via Freedom of Information Act requests."

11. Kennedy, Robert F. Jr., *The Real Anthony Fauci: Bill Gates, Big Pharma, and the Global War on Democracy* (New York: Skyhorse, due Nov. 9 2021)
12. Nussbaum, Bruce, *Good Intentions*, p. 122.
13. Lest anyone should think that FDA targets only gay men with AIDS for its deadly delays, rest assured they are equal opportunity delayers. Mary Ruwart reviews many of their deadly delays in *Death by Regulation* (San Francisco: Sun Star Press. 2018). See particularly her account of FDA's 20-year obstruction of information on folic acid used to prevent deadly spinal birth defects, pp 163-165.
14. Nussbaum, *Good Intentions*, p. 242.
15. See Driscoll, James, *How AIDS Activists Challenged America*, pp 77-116, details the activist struggle over underground ddC in which Driscoll and Delaney were the two major players. For an account written more from Delaney's point of view see, Jonathan Kwitney, *Acceptable Risks* (New York: Simon & Schuster,1991).
16. Driscoll, James, *How AIDS Activists Challenged America*, pp. 167-210.
17. Nussbaum, Bruce p. 125.
18. See "A Day in the Life of Dr. Anthony Fauci, Huffington Post, 12/3/20:
"What does one of the top infectious disease experts do when he's sidelined by the White House during COVID-19? Plenty. Here's what Fauci's thanksgiving eve looked like:
5:10 a.m. to 6 a.m. Showered and shaved
6 a.m. to 6:30 a.m. Resumed dealing with email
6:30 a.m. to 7 a.m. Appeared on ABC News' "Good Morning America"
7 a.m. to 7:30 a.m. Left home for NIH
7:30 a.m. to 8 a.m. Appeared on C-SPAN's "Washington Journal"
8 a.m. to 8:30 a.m. Appeared on WNYC-FM's "The Takeaway"
8:30 a.m. to 9 a.m. Interview with Chicago television station
9 a.m. to 10 a.m. Visited two COVID-19 patients under treatment at the NIH Clinical Center and their primary physicians
10 a.m. to 10:30 a.m. Video meeting with senior National Institute of Allergy and Infectious Diseases staff
10:30 a.m. to 11:00 a.m. Interview with newspaper reporter
11:00 a.m. to 11:50 a.m. Video meeting with Health and Human Services Secretary Alex Azar, NIH Director Francis Collins, CDC Director Robert Redford.
11:50 a.m. to 12 p.m. A bathroom break and more email
12 p.m. to 12:30 p.m. Interviewed with Byron Allen for the Grio on skepticism about the vaccine among Black Americans "

12:30 p.m. to 1 p.m. HuffPost interview #

1 p.m. to 1:30 p.m. Another television appearance

1:30 p.m. to 1:50 p.m. The elusive scheduled break $

1:50 p.m. to 2:30 p.m. Another newspaper interview %

2:30 p.m. to 3 p.m. Interview with scientific journal

3 p.m.... This continues on for hours until Fauci, "can no longer keep his eyes open."

19. For recent book length reviews critical of Fauci's use of science see: Berenson, Alex, *Unreported Truths about Covid 19 and Lockdowns* (Kindle, June 2021) Greer, Steven, *Tony's Virus: How Tony Fauci Became the Most Powerful Man in the World by Exploiting a Pandemic* (Independently published, Sept., 2020); Mikovits, Judy, *A Plague of Corruption*, (New York, Skyhorse , April 2020); Ortleb, Charles, *The Chronic Fatigue Syndrome Epidemic Cover-up,* (New York: CreateSpace, 2018).

20. Popper, Karl Raimund, *The Logic of Scientific Discovery* (London: Routledge, 2002) p 45.

21. The most comprehensive current source for information on ivermectin and other treatment and prevention protocols for Covid 19 is probably the FLCCC Alliance website (covid19criticalcare.com). The amount of online material on alternative therapies for Covid 19 is vast despite FDA efforts at suppression and censorship. One could write a much longer book than my current effort on this subject alone, so rather than attempt to summarize, I will suggest that the reader go online and explore.

22. Nearly all drugs have some safety issues for some people, as do in fact most foods. The safety issues for a number of common drugs, including aspirin and Tylenol, are in fact more serious and more common than those for the low dose short duration regimen of hydroxychloroquine used for Covid. With any safety concern, the keys are always the likelihood and possible seriousness of occurrences.

23. European regulators moved faster than FDA on approving thalidomide, as a result many more babies with the deformities were born there. The estimate for UK is more than 2000 babies. FDA moved more slowly on thalidomide approval and so largely avoided the disaster in the US. Why did FDA move more slowly? It was not greater caution of thoroughness the delayed FDA, thalidomide was delayed here simply because Francis Kelsey, the officer in charge, had taken several months of medical leave.

24. The parable of the talents, one of Jesus's most detailed parables, is largely forgotten today. However, English Reformation thinkers, particularly Shakespeare and Milton, drew important economic lessons from it. They saw the parable as giving economic activity a moral dimension it lacked for Medieval Catholics. Their approach is similar to that of contemporary Jungian thinkers who stress the soul making aspects of economic activity.

25. Oxfam International (website) May 20/2021. "Covid vaccines create nine new billionaires."

26. Meijer, Raul Ilargi, *Automatic Earth* (website) Jan 27, 2021.
27. Ruwart, Mary, p. 164.
28. Federal regulations exclude accelerated development of therapeutics for conditions that already have approved treatments. So, it was argued that if ivermectin were approved for Covid, then vaccines could not be developed on an accelerated basis. These regulations, however, might have been waived by executive order or an act of Congress.
29. Senator Marco Rubio, "Dr. Fauci lied about Coronavirus to Manipulate our behavior." Fox News Report, Dec. 30/2020/
30. Suderman, Peter, "The Pandemic Could Have Been Over Sooner if no for FDA." *Reason*, 5/19/2021.
31. Bernstein, Brittany, "Fauci Argued Benefits of Gain of Function Research Outweighed Pandemic Risk" *National Review*, 5/28/21.
32. Ainsley, Julia, "18 Percent of Migrant Families . . .," NBC News Online, 8/7/2021.
33. Hanson, Joseph Davis, "The Genesis of our Collective American Meltdown." *American Greatness*, 7/4/2021.
34. Codevilla, Angelo uses satire to put Babbitt's death in a broader socio-political perspective in, "Why Not Award Ashli Babbitt's Killer the Medal of Honor," *American Greatness*, 8/22/2021.
35. Sartre, Jean Paul, *Anti-Semite and Jew*, trans. George Becker (New York: Schocken, 1967) pp. 18-31.
36. Immanuel School, where Karen Pence teaches and where the Pences sent their children, proudly bases its anti LGBT policies on Leviticus 20:13: --- *"If a man lies with a male as with a woman, both of them have committed an abomination; they shall surely be put to death."* If the Pences' school's anti LGBT discrimination policies are any evidence, the school appears to believe that barbaric verse holds a place in Christian doctrine superior to the Sermon on the Mount.
37. Driscoll, James *How AIDS Activists Challenged America,* pp.239-246, recounts the AIDS community efforts behind persuading President Bush to take the unprecedented step of over-ruling the FDA by waiving their obstructive rules around HIV rapid testing. Bush's action should be credited with saving thousands of lives and reducing new cases of HIV by more than 15,000 per year.
38. In contemporary American society all deep dyed left wing opportunists become "Marxists for the day" when doing so allows them to take advantage of the new opportunities each new crisis presents.
39. See "Special Report: The stimulations driving the world's responses to Covid 19," *Nature*, 03/4/2020; also see, "How the UK government misrepresented Covid projections—explained, *The Guardian*, 11/6/2020.
40. See Joel Kotkin and Hugo Kruger, "The Coming Collapse of the Developing World," *Spiked* 7/23/2021. Kotkin and Kruger argue that by far the greatest damage and ultimately the greatest number of deaths due to Covid will not be from Covid itself but from a Covid panic induced economic collapse in

the developing world. One may speculate further that the damage from Covid induced political chaos will further amplify and ultimately dwarf even the direct economic damage.

41. See Driscoll, James, "The Lesson of Coronavirus: Re-invent FDA," *Washington Examiner*, May 8, 2020 which summarizes FDA's flubs early in the epidemic: *First, the FDA ordered Seattle researchers to halt testing because their lab was not certified. The agency also rejected available foreign paradigms to develop the FDA and the Centers for Disease Control and Prevention's own in-house tests, all the while forbidding private U.S. labs to initiate testing independently. But then, the first FDA-CDC tests had defective reagents. As if that weren't enough, the FDA waited two months to lift restrictions on tests from private labs, delayed the sale of home tests, and delayed masks and protective gear. Thanks mainly to the FDA, the U.S. response was bogged down until we passed the point where it was possible to contain the epidemic as South Korea did with its swift, flexible response. Today, supplies of masks and tests, including those for immunity, remain inadequate given demand.*

42. See Jordan, Jim, "What Did Fauci Know and When? His Emails Point to Panic, Lies, and a Possible Cover-up," *Federalist* 7/14/21.

43. The bad record of the safety protocols in the Wuhan lab is often cited in defense of the view that the release of the virus was accidental. What helps let the Chinese off the hook puts Fauci back on the hook. Why, we must ask, would he want to fund gain of function research that he knew to be extremely dangerous at a lab whose safety precautions were known to be deficient?

44. For a good recent survey on the efficacy of masking see, Jeffrey Anderson, *City Journal*, 8/11/21. Anderson concludes:
In sum, of the 14 RCTs that have tested the effectiveness of masks in preventing the transmission of respiratory viruses, three suggest, but do not provide any statistically significant evidence in intention-to-treat analysis, that masks might be useful. The other eleven suggest that masks are either useless—whether compared with no masks or because they appear not to add to good hand hygiene alone—or actually counterproductive. Of the three studies that provided statistically significant evidence in intention-to-treat analysis that was not contradicted within the same study, one found that the combination of surgical masks and hand hygiene was less effective than hand hygiene alone, one found that the combination of surgical masks and hand hygiene was less effective than nothing, and one found that cloth masks were less effective than surgical masks. Hiram Powers, the nineteenth-century neoclassical sculptor, keenly observed, "The eye is the window to the soul, the mouth the door. The intellect, the will, are seen in the eye; the emotions, sensibilities, and affections, in the mouth." The best available scientific evidence suggests that the American people, credulously trusting their public-health officials, have been blocking the door to the soul without blocking the transmission of the novel coronavirus.

45. See "Redfield: Covid 19 was in Wuhan in September or October 2019.

Medpage Today, 3/29/2021.

46. Wallace-Wells, David, "On the Risk to Kids," *New York Mag.* 7/12/ 2021

47. *In the UK "Five Times More Children Committed Suicide During Covid Lockdown than Died of Covid: UK Study," Epoch Times, 8/15/ 2021. Spotty information reveals similar disparities in other countries including the US. Only right wing press, like Fox News, appears to be covering this very significant story. In my home town of Las Vegas, school lockdowns were relaxed because of news of a big spike in student suicides.. Unfortunately, this got little national coverage.*

48. Bureaucrats and politicians, not unlike scientists, follow the patterns adjustment/resistance to change outlined by Thomas Kuhns in *The Structure of Scientific Revolutions*, (Chicago: Univ. of Chicago Press, 1996).

49. Dr. Francis Kelsey, the FDA officer in charge of processing the thalidomide NDA, was on medical leave for several months at the time. Insiders have told me that her leave, rather than any special precautions on the part of FDA, delayed the approval procedure long enough for the deformities to begin showing up in UK and other places where thalidomide was approved earlier.

50. See Ruwart, 41-42, 131-137.

51. For another critical review of FDA abuses and the need to major agency reforms, see Henry Miller, *To America's Health: A Proposal to Reform the Food and Drug Administration,* (Palo Alto, Ca., Hoover Institution Press, 2013). Despite a general consensus that FDA reform is definitely needed that prevails the right and extends into the political middle, surprisingly little has been published outlining specific plans or programs for FDA reform.

52. Ruwart, p. 142.

Index

CPSIA information can be obtained
at www.ICGtesting.com
Printed in the USA
JSHW051534040122
21771JS00006B/164